MISSION POSSIBLE

PAVING THE ROAD TO UNIVERSAL HEALTH COVERAGE

SWAMI SUBRAMANIAM
APARAJITHAN SRIVATHSAN

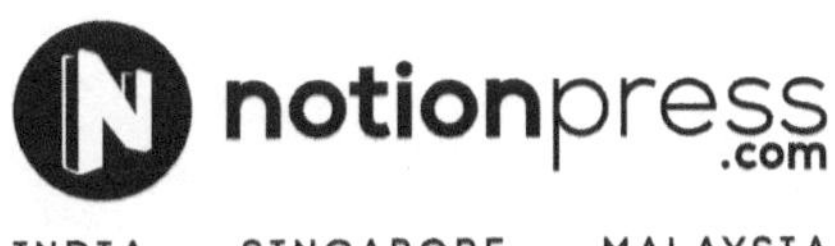

ISBN 979-8-89186-388-0

Universal health coverage means that all people have access to the full range of quality health services they need, when and where they need them, without financial hardship. It covers the full continuum of essential health services, from health promotion to prevention, treatment, rehabilitation and palliative care. - *World Health Organization*

The issue of universal coverage is not a matter of economics. Little more than 1 percent of GDP assigned to health could cover all. It is a matter of soul. - *Uwe Reinhardt*

We dedicate this book to the millions of Indians who suffer from a lack of affordable and quality healthcare. We hope this book stimulates the conversations and drives the actions that will end their suffering.

Praise for Mission Possible (continued from back cover)

"Mission Possible" makes a strong and persuasive argument for Universal Health Care based on the foundations of a resilient and strong primary health care system. Written in an easily understandable style without needless data and jargon, the book provides several suggestions as to how India might consider different models for ensuring efficient and affordable health care within a mixed system of delivery where both public and private sector work together. The message that only a dominant tax based financing with government as the lead stakeholder can ensure an inclusive and equitable system of care comes out loud and clear. It is an interesting book furthering the debate for a more caring and inclusive health system and worth a read.

Kanuru Sujatha Rao, Former Secretary,
Ministry of Health, Government of India

The healthcare scenario has changed a lot in the past few years, due to massive developments in technology, and the unscrupulous commercialization of Healthcare. It is evident that a balance between primary, secondary and tertiary care is essential to achieve UHC. However, the book 'Mission Possible' brings new, comprehensive, and necessary value addition to the road towards UHC. This book is logical, evidenced based and easy to read.

Rev. Dr. Mathew Abraham, Director General,
The Catholic Health Association of India

This book has taken a complex issue and delved into each lever that has either a positive or a negative influence. A paradigm shift in thinking and allowing time for newer ways of healthcare delivery to take its roots needs committed leadership at the political, executive and provider level. As a practicing health care professional this book educated me on the macro and micro factors that have an influence on healthcare delivery. Universal Health Coverage is the Holy Grail that has been elusive for too long. Having this solid road map and a willingness to genuinely try is what is the need of the hour. Thank you for having the courage and conviction to address such a complex problem.

Dr. S Aravind, Chief Medical Officer, Aravind Eye Hospital

The holy grail of healthcare is to achieve universal coverage that can make quality healthcare affordable and accessible to all irrespective of their geographic location or economic status. For a long time, this has been assumed to be "Mission Impossible." This book, aptly titled "Mission Possible" analyzes the entire healthcare ecosystem to say why Universal Health Coverage may not be beyond our means.

Dr. Sumanth Raman, medical professional,
television and media personality, author, and founder of Algorithm Health

CONTENTS

ABBREVIATIONS

Bio	Billion
CCC	Comprehensive Care Center
CCP	Comprehensive Care Physician
CHW	Community Health Worker
DALY	Disability Adjusted Life years
EHR	Electronic Health Record
FHF	Focused Healthcare Factory
GH	General Hospital
GP	General Practitioner
HIP	Health Innovation Park
HIS	Health Information Systems
IT	Information technology
Mil	Million
NCD	Non-communicable disease
NHS	National Health Service (UK)
OPD	Outpatient Department
PHC	Primary Health Center
RoI	Return on Investment
THW	Tech-enabled Health Worker
UHC	Universal Health Coverage
WaFEr	Waste, Fraud, and Error
YLD	Years of life lost due to disability
YLL	Years of life lost

PREFACE

India is at a crossroads with regard to its health system. Doing nothing is not an option. While still at an early stage of health system development and spending, India needs to avoid entrenching a high-cost, low-value delivery system. If the economy slows, health spending will probably not follow suit. An aging population and demands for hospital care and new technologies will continue to exert upward cost pressures. If current trends hold, India's future generations will likely inherit an expensive health system that provides little value for money, fails to deliver improved patient health, and undermines economic growth.

– Niti Aayog

India can no longer tolerate the paradox in which child mortality and under-nutrition rates are worse than in many poorer nations, in which women face an unrelenting burden of unsafe childbirth, and in which communicable diseases, mental disorders, chronic diseases, and injuries prevent people from leading healthy lives. India can no longer accept a healthcare system that is frequently exploitative, almost completely unregulated, and so poorly performing. The health conditions for most have to improve if all Indians want to enjoy the freedoms that lend value to their lives. A healthy India is also crucial for the country to make the most of its demographic advantage and to sustain economic prosperity.

– Patel V et al., Universal health care in India: the time is right
Lancet, 2011

The two Indias

Where healthcare is concerned, there are two Indias. There is the India of the rich: citizens who have private insurance and on-demand access to healthcare. And then there is the much larger India, which relies on creaky and dysfunctional public institutions that barely cover rudimentary healthcare needs. India was ranked 145th among 195 countries in the 2018 Healthcare Access and Quality Index. On almost any health indicator, India is middling in performance, if not a downright laggard, even compared to our South Asian neighbors. It is not as if India has not made strides in healthcare. For example, in communicable diseases, India has achieved a 71% reduction in disability-adjusted life years (DALYs, defined as years of productive life lost due to illness per lakh population) between 1991 and 2019. It is quite another thing that both China (starting from a smaller base in 1991) and Bangladesh (starting from a larger base in 1991) have witnessed an over 82% reduction in DALYs due to communicable diseases in the same period. Bangladesh's absolute incidence of communicable disease per lakh population in 2019 (at 6,903) is below India's (at 9,438).

Fixing Healthcare

It is neither ethical nor consistent with good government to have a two-track system of healthcare—one for the rich and another for the poor. There is also a practical reason to focus on this issue—if we do not bring down levels of illness in the population, then productivity will be affected and the much-touted demographic dividend will disappear. Policymakers have periodically produced comprehensive reports on what needs to be done. Unfortunately, policymakers have not implemented the sensible and common-sense suggestions presented in these reports. If the Bhore Committee Report (1946)[1] had been followed in letter and spirit, we may not have been in the situation in which we are today. In 1962, the Mudaliar Committee report[2] said, "... the new Primary Health Centers to be opened should be on the pattern of the recommendations of the Bhore Committee … to serve a population of up to 40,000 … and curative, preventive, and promotive services should all be provided at the PHC." The Mudaliar Committee also recommended that an All-India Health service should be created to replace the erstwhile Indian Medical service. Successive Governments ignored both these recommendations, only paying lip service to healthcare. Despite grand announcements in budget speeches, when it came to implementation, Governments tinkered half-heartedly.

Hopefully, this will change. Three decades into India's economic liberalization, the realization has dawned that our economic destiny is tightly coupled to the health of our citizens. Universal Health Coverage is a topic that is extensively covered in mainstream media, and politicians are giving it the attention it deserves. But this has not triggered serious debate as to which model of Universal Health Coverage will work for India and how we can get there from where we are today. It would be foolish to assume a desired end state in the future without accounting for the social and technological forces that will buffet healthcare along the way. The aging population and the introduction of expensive new healthcare technologies mean that the model for healthcare delivery cannot simply be a scaled-up version of what we have today. We must not only front-load analysis of trends, but we also need to keep revisiting the models derived from such analysis to ensure that they remain in sync with evolving reality. This is especially important in the case of emerging technologies like cell therapy and artificial intelligence. The full play of such developments, even as they continue to evolve and surprise us, cannot be determined with precision.

Even as India makes progress through mission-mode public health initiatives in controlling communicable diseases, a much more dangerous enemy in the form of non-communicable disease stalks the country. From 1991 to 2019, even as communicable disease DALYs decreased by 71%, non-communicable (NCD) disease DALYs increased by 13.9%. Given the ongoing epidemic rise of obesity and diabetes, DALYs due to NCDs will grow even faster in the future. There is an obvious need to provide an active screening-driven primary prevention and chronic disease control program that addresses the major killers—hypertension, diabetes, stroke, heart disease, chronic obstructive pulmonary disease, and common cancers. This is the role of primary healthcare. There is no doubting the importance of good primary healthcare. It has to be the bedrock on which Universal Health Coverage is established. But even in primary healthcare it cannot be business as usual. New models adapted to current realities will have to be invented.

Laissez-faire Will Not Do

Why not let things evolve organically as the marketplace grows and evolves? For the reasons enumerated below, such a laissez-faire attitude is unlikely to provide sustainable and equitable solutions.

Healthcare is not just another business. It is an essential commodity. In a fair and just society, everyone must have access to quality healthcare. We have drifted away from this ideal. A common notion is that private for-profit investment in healthcare will bring efficiency and quality. The real backstory is that in opaque fee-for-service healthcare, the buyer has no control or choice over the decision to buy. This is compounded by the fact that, unlike efficient markets in which multiple players can compete on equal terms to serve the customer, healthcare delivery tends to be hyper-local. It is hard for new players to penetrate a market where there is a single player with a dominant market share. As a result, the sellers' motive to increase income by driving increased consumption goes unchecked. On top of this, the profit motive causes a catalytic and runaway explosion in prices. At the same time, quality gets short shrift since it is a much harder signal for the consumer to track—for example, consumers do not have access to data on the comparative success rates for the same treatment at different hospitals.

Governments have mistakenly subscribed to the notion that corporate healthcare can be a substitute for public healthcare. Growth in private healthcare, fanned by a mix of deliberate policy and benign neglect, has only led to the proliferation of expensive hospitals catering to the rich at prices that are not affordable for the rest. Optimization happens, but it is an optimization of profits and not optimization of affordability or quality.

The test for Indian policymakers and politicians will be their ability to chart a route to Universal Health Coverage (UHC) that deftly navigates the minefields *en route*. The ability of policymakers and politicians to make the tough decisions needed to reach UHC is unproven and untested. If protests against the farm laws are any indication, then it is likely that sections of civil society will also challenge the trade-offs needed as part of a move toward UHC. To ensure wide acceptance, the transition must be painless. This will require leaders to understand the options and translate the choices in simple ways to the voter. They must put in the work to figure out which choices (at least *a priori*) make the most sense. They must avoid getting bogged down in ideological sand traps and have the flexibility to allow fresh evidence from experience to inform and influence the choices. This means we will need infrastructure, programs, and processes specifically built to experiment safely with alternate models before deciding which model is ready to be scaled up for all 1.4 billion Indians.

Thinking Heads: Commissions and Committees

The British medical journal Lancet has commissioned a group of experts: 'the Lancet Citizens' Commission on re-imagining India's health system[3] to lay out the path to achieving UHC in India in the coming decade. A guiding principle for this Commission is - "structural change toward UHC can only be attained through consultative and participatory engagement with the diverse sectors involved in healthcare and with India's citizenry...to formulate a road map for realizing a resilient health system that offers comprehensive, accountable, accessible, inclusive, and affordable quality healthcare ... with a focus ... on the architecture of India's health system." It is to be expected that they will focus their attention on figuring out and recommending ways to prevent illness in the midst of India's demographic transition. This will be a natural emphasis for any comprehensive appraisal of the healthcare system we need to build. While the bias is warranted, it should not overshadow equally important analysis and weighing of choices in tertiary healthcare. It is where at least 40% of expenditure on healthcare occurs. Improving the efficiency and productivity of our hospitals will free up resources that can be redirected toward primary and preventive health.

Cooperative efforts of this kind, which assemble groups of influential individuals, are necessarily consultative. Such committees have a tendency to avoid formulations that can be perceived as controversial or extreme. The averaging of opinions results in a watered-down set of recommendations. While we are broadly aligned with the mission of the Lancet Commission, we have also used our freedom as individuals to push the envelope. We are emphatic in our belief that healthcare has to undergo radical transformation if Universal Health Coverage is to become feasible. We provide several examples of radical transformation—including a completely new vision for Primary Healthcare, so radical in its ambit that we propose a name change, calling it Comprehensive Care. Another is the idea of "focused care hospitals" as a means to produce quality healthcare at an affordable cost. We are also quite definitive in recommending much more proactive involvement by the Government in bringing about these transformations.

Committee-led or federated approaches also tend to get bogged down in the process, which means the output gets delayed. An example of a federated approach was the Swasth Alliance (swasthalliance.org) - an alliance of 150 organizations, which was formed to address the COVID-19 pandemic. The initial pandemic-driven enthusiasm lost steam once the pandemic waned, and an ambitious plan for the creation of a National Medical Oxygen Grid has not been implemented. It has subsequently redirected its efforts toward creating the architecture for a "health claims exchange." In the section on health technology, we call for stewardship by the Government in the development and deployment of health innovation. Both the Lancet Commission and the Swasth Alliance lack formal Government support. Government involvement can be a mixed blessing. But in healthcare, it is necessary. Without Government support, decentralized innovation models will not succeed in healthcare.

There is a danger of being excessively anchored in today's reality. This results in a timid approach that avoids rocking the boat. We hope that the Lancet Commission and other collective healthcare policy think tanks will create an impact on healthcare by delivering powerful, transforming, and definitive recommendations. Even if the implementation of radical change has to be staggered to avoid major dislocation, it is important to recognize the most desirable end state and pave the path toward that.

What the pandemic (has not) taught us

While the pandemic has refocused public attention on healthcare, particularly hospital care, the pandemic experience cannot inform us about the healthcare we need. Even if pandemics become common, they will remain less frequent than the bread-and-butter illnesses that plague our population. While we present our views on how hospitals can be strengthened for mass hospitalization events, the deep structural changes we recommend are not conditioned by the pandemic experience. In one way, though, the pandemic has helped. It has engendered dissatisfaction with the existing situation and triggered soul-searching debates of the kind that are needed if we are to build a new healthcare system.

Why did we write this book?

We are at a critical inflection point for Indian healthcare. Growth in income has raised the capacity of the average citizen to pay for healthcare. But this has been overshadowed by the growth in the cost of healthcare and the epidemic spread of lifestyle disorders. In the coming years, there will be significant stress in the system to equitably and affordably satisfy demand. While disease prevention, public health, and primary healthcare will remain cornerstones in any national strategy, we should not be blind to the need to cater to the upsurge in demand for tertiary care in complex hospital environments. Our national aspiration of Universal Health Coverage is now on the front burner. This is an optimal time to discuss and develop strategies that will work to get us closer to this aspiration. This book is an attempt to stimulate a conversation on a topic that affects us all.

We must also pause and think of the course of events that might befall us if we do not take steps now. An explosion in non-communicable disease[4] overlaid with periodic eruptions of climate change-driven pandemics can decimate productivity and stunt our economy. A surge in out-of-pocket expenditure on catastrophic illnesses will leave a significant proportion of the population impoverished, and the rest without savings needed for major lifetime expenses like education and retirement. The rates for cardiovascular disease have seen a 34% increase between 1990 and 2016, and healthcare cost inflation ticks up at a 14% annual rate. If we put those numbers together, we can imagine the untenable crisis that will emerge, as early as 2050.

There is plenty of hand-wringing around healthcare, not just in India, but everywhere in the world. However, practical solutions are rarely aired. Perhaps because many commentators balk at the enormity of the task. Proposals that seek to dislodge existing players and systems may sound like pipe dreams. But we have no choice in the matter. This is not a moment for cosmetic surgery. We have to do radical surgery, even if it means lopping off and reconstructing key components in order to save the system as a whole. We view this book as a manifesto for a viable and practical system of healthcare that meets the objectives of Universal Health Coverage. Better healthcare is within our means. But actions have to be initiated now.

Our Audience

This book is aimed at an audience consisting of policymakers, private healthcare delivery companies, healthcare activists, politicians, and members of civil society concerned about healthcare delivery in India.

The middle class in India plays a role in our elections that belies their size. They are articulate, educated, and have the disposable income needed to make their voices heard. Unfortunately, they have shown apathy when it comes to healthcare. In the past, healthcare has been a relatively small proportion of the middle-class family budget. This has changed. Even the middle class is starting to feel the pinch of out-of-pocket expenses and insurance premiums. As a result, they have started engaging with the system to determine what is best for them at an individual level. But their collective voices must speak out for the nation as a whole, and not just for themselves. We address this book to this vibrant constituency. An engaged and informed middle class can play the role of interlocutor between citizens and the people who govern. The material in this book will help them inform themselves so that they can drive the right choices for the nation through the ballot box. Eventually, if Government initiatives to push governance of local health systems into local communities through bodies like the "Rogi Kalyan Samities" spread, then this book (translated into Indian languages) can serve as a thought platform from which new ideas to improve healthcare delivery can blossom.

Narrative Structure

Books of this genre tend to be heavy on data and analysis. This book is too. But we go further to make inferences based on the data we accessed, some of which are summarized in the tables we have assembled and presented at the back of this book. From these inferences, we derive a prescription for an architecture for Universal Health Coverage in India. We have interviewed many stakeholders and reviewed the results of experiments done globally in the provision of UHC. From the insights based on this research, we have developed our thesis about how UHC can be achieved in India. We have not hesitated to take the plunge and provide a prescription; waffling on this would not have been helpful to those hoping to gain a new perspective from this book. While we have in many instances aligned with wisdom generated in other countries, we have tailored our prescriptions to suit India.

This has not been an easy book to write. If we look at the many microcosms and moving parts within healthcare, then we find that the most optimal solution for one part can be sub-optimal for another. Trade-offs have to be made. Our approach has been to take a system-wide view and optimize prescriptions for the whole system rather than for pieces. This runs against the prevailing system of healthcare, whose fragmented character causes each piece to optimize for itself without considering the knock-on effects on other parts of the ecosystem. By considering the system as a whole, we discovered opportunities where the net benefit to the patient vastly outweighs any downsides of system-wide optimization.

The book is organized into four sections. Each section focuses on a particular aspect of healthcare. The pieces within each section appear as chapters, many of which, in earlier versions, have seen the light of day in newspaper articles and magazines. Our approach is not simply to catalog and describe a problem. We have applied ourselves to proposing solutions. Despite the daunting complexity and magnitude of the challenges in healthcare, we are convinced that scalable and simple interventions along with structural changes can effectively solve the principal challenges. We have dissected key leverage points that can have catalytic benefits. We also take the view that the ugly aspects of healthcare, such as rampant waste, fraud, and error, can be viewed positively as opportunities for correction that will free up resources. In the last section, we summarize the interventions that can serve as a starting point for us to build the healthcare system we need. This is not an academic text; however, we have included references and readings in support of the contestable points we make. We have also added fifteen tables at the end that give a panoramic view of healthcare from an Indian perspective. We have included commentary on the tables to draw attention to data that informs the debate on UHC.

We hope this book will inform your perspective on what needs to be done. Even if you find some of the points we make contestable, we hope you will engage with the ideas and refresh your thinking. Our collective engagement on this topic as Indians is vital if our goal of providing high-quality healthcare to ALL Indians is to be realized in the coming decades.

THE ECOSYSTEM

To bring about transformational change in healthcare, tinkering at the edges will not be sufficient. The entire Ecosystem must be considered, starting with a new vision for primary care to how we should re-engineer the provision of tertiary care. As an integral component of this vision, we also outline new structures and ways of working, including upturning traditional hierarchies in the healthcare workforce.

A new approach to primary health care is central to achieving the SDGs and UHC. Progress will require courage and determination, but the time is right. The world has never been better positioned for success.

A Vision for Primary Health Care in the 21st Century (Technical Series, WHO and UNICEF)

The conventional factory attempts to do too many conflicting production tasks within one inconsistent set of manufacturing policies. The chief result is that the plant is likely to be non-competitive because its policies are not focused on the one key manufacturing task essential to successfully competing in its industry.

Wickham Skinner, The Focused Factory, Harvard Business Review (1974)

If money were no object, we might all enjoy what has been described as "presidential medicine", a one-to-one relationship with our physician. But since the allocation of scarce resources is an ever-present reality, the question increasingly arises: How many doctors are enough?

Jeffrey E. Harris in "How many doctors are enough?" Health Affairs (1986)

The doctors may be mapping out the war games, but it is the nurses who make the conflict bearable.

Jodi Picoult, an American writer

01 | WHY WE NEED TO CONSIDER THE WHOLE ECOSYSTEM

People experience illnesses in episodes. Each episode can influence the subsequent trajectory of health. Failed management of hypertension or diabetes in youth can cause kidney damage, requiring hospitalization later in life. Likewise, cesarean childbirth can affect the child's health when it grows into an adult.

Because of these inter-dependencies, we should not prioritize one aspect of healthcare without understanding the trade-offs. Healthcare decisions must not only consider today's costs and benefits but also the lifetime costs and benefits of the choices made. Tight control of blood glucose with the aid of continuous glucose monitoring is expensive, but worthwhile if it prevents kidney failure. However, tight glucose monitoring and control in an eighty-year-old can increase the likelihood of dangerously low blood glucose compared to the tiny marginal utility of preventing diabetes complications at that age.

The inter-dependencies also apply at a systems level. For example, the budget for healthcare is a zero-sum game. If we spend more on hospitals, less money will be available for primary care. Similarly, if more doctors decide to practice specialty medicine in hospitals there will be fewer doctors available to deliver primary care.

Each piece of healthcare has varying levels of complexity, costs, value, and difficulty in execution. Changing behavior—for example, stopping smoking or eating healthy food—can be hard to accomplish but least complex to deliver. Such interventions also have low short-term but high long-term value, for example by preventing a stroke or heart attack several decades later. They also cost less. On the other hand, a coronary bypass in later life has predictable immediate outcomes, although it is complex to deliver, is expensive, and delivers most of its value in the short to medium term. Balancing these issues to determine where we ought to invest and where we can allow unmet needs requires a whole-system, whole-life approach to healthcare.

Depending on where we are with respect to the healthcare ecosystem, we get a different view, just like the blind men who each tried to describe an elephant based on the part they touched. The healthcare worker sees the inner workings of the system. Insurance companies see the payment mechanisms and their own role in enabling them. The Government sees its delivery systems, the population as a whole, and the pieces it regulates tightly. The patient sees only the clinic, the hospital, the diagnostic laboratory, the pharmacy where she goes to access healthcare. This fragmentation is exacerbated by specialty based care, with different specialist physicians calling the shots for different illnesses. But none of these individual pieces operate in isolation. Performance improvements in one component can worsen performance elsewhere. For example, discharging patients sooner after a hospitalization event may save money now but increase the chances of readmission for the same condition, thus nullifying the savings from early discharge.

The multiplicity of components that constitute healthcare create inherent centrifugal forces when the individual components are not coordinated. Opportunistic private providers focus on the most commercially attractive pieces of the healthcare pie without taking into view upstream and downstream consequences. For example, a hospital that performs angioplasty for coronary heart disease may not invest the time and effort needed for post-procedure cardiac rehabilitation, because that line of business is not as profitable. As a result, patients suffer a high rate of relapse requiring re-hospitalization. For the hospital, such re-hospitalization is revenue accretive, and there is no incentive to change. Similarly, cardiologists may not spend time counseling patients on nutritional approaches to preventing heart disease since the consultation fee is fixed regardless of the time spent with the patient. Such moral hazards abound in healthcare. Individual players take actions that are in their self-interest, resulting in increased costs and lowered quality.

"Wicked Problems" are best solved by applying "Design Thinking."

The design theorist Horst Rittel is credited with coining the term "Wicked Problem" for problems that are multidimensional and complex[1]. Given the multiplicity of the components of healthcare: from home care to the hospital, from elective to emergency care, and from prevention to curative care, each with its own stakeholders, the problem of integration in healthcare is exquisitely complex and qualifies as a "wicked problem".

The "Wicked" nature of problems in healthcare has also been articulated as the Iron Triangle: Access, Affordability, and Quality form three sides of the Iron Triangle[2]. For example, it is possible to improve any two of the sides of the Triangle, but it will have to come at the cost of compromising the third side of the Triangle. For example, if you increase Quality by deploying personnel with more experience, then the higher salaries you have to pay them will increase the cost of care, thus diminishing affordability. If you attempt to increase affordability by concentrating physical resources like hospitals in fewer locations, then you will reduce access for some segments of the population that live far away.

The cognitive scientist Herbert Simon came up with the concept of "Design Thinking" as a way to find solutions to such wicked problems[3]. "Design Thinking" is a set of principles that are applied to the process of finding the optimal solution. It uses an iterative prototyping process that is focused on the user experience. In the case of healthcare, it is the patient and not the healthcare worker whose preferences should be given priority during design.

The "Design Thinking" approach is consumer-centric and holistic, with empathy for consumer needs. It takes a longitudinal rather than episodic view of the provider-consumer relationship. So, on the one hand, Design Thinking can help solve problems and improve performance in healthcare delivery by creating processes and tools that help the provider improve efficiency and quality. On the other hand, it can also improve patient experience by creating processes wrapped around their needs, instead of bending their needs to suit the process. Such design principles are critical in the development and deployment of services and procedures close to or in the home of the patient, and for seamless vertical integration of care from home to hospital and back. "Design Thinking" brings the focus back on patient needs rather than provider preference.

While the Iron Triangle of healthcare plays out as expected in most scenarios, we can think of exceptions that break "the strangle of the Iron Triangle." For example, can we increase quality and lower costs at the same time without compromising access? We may not achieve this within any isolated piece of the healthcare ecosystem, but we may be able to achieve this with the whole ecosystem, i.e. a loss to one part of the system may be more than compensated by a gain elsewhere. This is also why we must consider and solve for the whole ecosystem from a patient perspective, rather than a piece of the ecosystem from the provider perspective. The thoughts laid out below are influenced by this thinking.

Both horizontal and vertical integration are necessary.

In most industries, horizontal integration within a narrow segment, for example, the acquisition of one automotive company by another, is desirable: it results in economies of scale, improved efficiency, and greater market power. In healthcare as well, increasing specialization within narrow areas (usually based on organ and age, e.g. pediatric cardiothoracic surgery) is the trend. However, patients expect to be treated as a whole and not merely as an assembly of organs. When illness affects more than one organ, as is often the case with seriously ill patients, specialists treating each organ have to engage in a complex dance of hand-offs which quickly degenerates into a game of Chinese whispers with the probability of error rising exponentially with each additional specialist who is brought in for the care of the patient. Often the hand-off does not even take place because the doctors do not have the time to talk to each other to share information. Integration of care across specialties is needed to fix this problem. Within the hospital environment, the role of a "hospitalist" has been created to fix this problem. A "hospitalist" is a generalist who is responsible for coordinating care across multiple specialities for a hospitalized patient.

A similar problem arises when the patient is first seen by a primary care physician and is then handed off to a specialist for advanced care. To eliminate this problem, we need vertical integration of care from the front-lines of care all the way back into tertiary or hospital-based care. Integration of care is not easy to manage or pull off in the classical for-profit scheme of things where each piece of healthcare is often in competition with other pieces for the healthcare rupee.

Vertical integration is achievable through a variety of means: a backbone structure that orchestrates the entirety of healthcare can be enabled through health-IT to maintain a one-truth record of the patient's health experience. Beyond the use use of tools like health-IT, total ownership of the patient's health journey in terms of control and accountability by a single agent like the primary care physician is what is needed to improve clinical outcomes. This is the structure we outline in the following section.

02 | PRIMARY HEALTHCARE

Commentaries on Universal Health Coverage emphasize the importance of primary healthcare as a foundational asset. However, most do not address two issues specifically: why is the current model retreating despite universal endorsement of its importance, and what substitute model of primary healthcare will succeed in its place. The assumption is that the traditional model of primary healthcare — which is currently moribund — can be revived. This, in our view, is a pipe dream. As Albert Einstein said, it is utter stupidity to keep doing the same old things and expect different results. In this section, we dissect the problem and propose a solution that will work.

We envision a model of primary healthcare that is very different from what we have today. We label it Comprehensive Care to distinguish it from legacy models of primary care. While sophisticated organ-based specialty care may have reduced primary care to the role of handmaiden, we see a need for robust primary care that serves as the backbone of healthcare, holding together all the disparate pieces. But first, what are the reasons for the failure of primary healthcare in its current form?

Primary healthcare is a broken "solution shop."

The clinical situations that primary healthcare has to deal with run the entire gamut of what can go wrong with someone's health. Since primary healthcare is the first stop for the patient, there is very little clinical history or records about the patient available to the doctor. Furthermore, primary care is expected to manage everything, from prevention of disease through lifestyle interventions, behavioral and mental health issues, issues resulting from poverty, disease management for non-communicable diseases, and coordination with specialist and tertiary care. The range of solutions that the primary care physician is expected to offer is extremely wide, spanning almost everything in medicine. Nothing is out of scope. The clinical issues in primary healthcare are classic examples of complex and unstructured problems.

The business model that responds to a complex and unstructured problem is called the "solution shop" model[4]. Primary care is a "solution shop" since it is meant to diagnose and solve unstructured problems. The automotive repair shop is an example of a "solution shop." When your car develops a problem, you go to the automotive shop, which is run by a generalist foreman who is broadly experienced in many aspects of automotive care. But he is not an expert on many of the details, for which he relies on a team of specialists. The first step is for the foreman with the help of his team to diagnose the problem. He then delegates work to specialists—a person who can fix radiator problems, another who fixes issues with the suspension, another who can do denting and painting, and yet another person who is good with electrical problems. The generalist foreman gets the work done in coordination with the appropriate specialist. And when the job is complete the foreman is the person who speaks to you and explains the bill and repairs done.

In our conception, the primary care physician should be like the auto shop foreman—a generalist who is overall in-charge. She is the person who marshals and deploys specialist resources as required for specific problems. Of course, medicine, as practiced today, is nothing like this. You meet the primary care physician who hands you off to a specialist, and when the specialist has finished his work, he may or may not (more often not) refer you back to the primary care doctor with a referral note explaining what was done, why it was done, and what follow-up care may be required. It is as though when you visit the auto shop, the foreman simply fobs you off to one of the technicians, forcing you to engage directly with 2 to 3 different technicians, none of whom coordinates work with the other technicians or with the foreman. Imagine how you would feel, as you are kicked around like a football. But this is exactly what happens in healthcare on a routine basis. This is a key problem we must solve if we are to evolve a model of healthcare that can deliver the goods.

Even as recently as the middle of the last century, primary care in the avatar of the family physician was at the center of the healthcare universe. The family doctor was the first port of call, and often the only port of call, since they were expected to manage everything from a boil to the delivery of a baby. And then, with the atomization of medicine came the unstoppable rise of medical specialties. The family doctor became the master of none—someone who is highly suspect in the eyes of demanding tech-savvy consumers, who are always on the lookout for the latest and the best. Corporate medicine was happy to step in and serve this consumer with all the gadgets that modern medicine could muster, but none of the heart that the family doctor used to offer.

Primary care saves lives but suffers from an existential crisis

Several studies have shown that good primary care can save costs and lives[5,6,7]. Specifically, the availability of good primary care was associated with lower mortality in the population being served, an increase in the delivery of high-value care, and higher patient-reported satisfaction. And yet, primary care as a specialty is in decline. You will be hard-pressed to find doctors who call themselves Primary Care Physicians or General Practitioners in India's metros. The only place where the primary care moniker still finds usage is in government-run primary health centers.

What is behind the decline in primary care? One is the increasing trend towards specialism in medicine. For every organ (heart, liver, kidney, brain, spine) and even for many diseases (diabetes, cancer) we have specialists. In the meantime, primary care physicians have seen a decline in their skills and the bandwidth of their capabilities. An encounter with a primary care physician often leads to a referral to a specialist physician. For the patient, this means having to deal with the inconvenience of two consultations, and therefore, they choose to take control and consult a specialist from the get-go. Like moths attracted to a flame, patients are attracted by the bells and whistles offered by specialty care, even for the most trivial ailment. They conflate specialty care with good healthcare and, as a result, they no longer want to be treated by a general practitioner.

The idea that an MBBS doctor will aspire to specialize in primary care is no longer true. Many doctors graduate with large debts. Even if the debt load is not large, their life aspirations cannot be met on the income of a primary care physician. To be a successful primary care physician, one needs to build a practice serving the same community over a lifetime. In today's world where people prefer mobility for a variety of reasons: spouse's occupation, children's education, etc., it is not possible to put down roots in any one community for the length of a lifetime.

The easy availability of specialists and hospital care in urban centers has decimated the ranks of primary care physicians. In the only place where primary healthcare is still delivered—the government primary health centers—the lack of medicines and equipment is compounded by rampant absenteeism among staff. The patients they are supposed to cater to have no faith in their ability to deliver. They either avoid seeing a doctor or wait long enough for the health issue to flare up. This is unfortunate since they end up dipping deeper into their paltry savings when they eventually take recourse to a private provider. In the absence of primary healthcare, there will be no one charged with preventing non-communicable diseases and their complications. The inevitable result will be unchecked growth in complications arising from untreated or under-treated non-communicable diseases. Without strong primary healthcare as the first port of call for patients, Universal Health Coverage will implode due to runaway costs.

Primary care needs re-masculation

Tinkering will not do; primary care in its current form is moribund and cannot serve the purpose of energizing UHC. We need a muscular version of primary healthcare as a response to a world where medicine has become more complex, more expensive, and more specialized. It has to be the counterfactual that works against the centrifugal tendencies that shred the healthcare experience. It must be the force that brings about a more responsive and patient-centric operational model to healthcare. At the same time, it must retain the virtues of the family doctor: easy access, convenience, and a lifelong relationship. In addition, it must acquire new virtues demanded by the modern-day healthcare consumer—it must be comprehensive, and serve as the front end for the entire gamut of the healthcare needs of a family. However, today's hyper-specialized medical system means that, inevitably, the patient will need to be referred to a specialist at some point in the healthcare journey. When this happens, there is a need for a patient-facing node in the delivery system to coordinate care through all the tangles and mazes that a patient with a complex condition has to navigate. Primary care has to be the glue that holds together the pieces of healthcare by providing such overarching coordination.

An ideal primary care delivery system should do this:

What should the 'perfect' primary healthcare system do? - We can start by quoting from the recommendations made in a National Academies consensus report[8]:

"1. Pay for primary care teams to care for people, not doctors to deliver services. 2. Ensure that high-quality primary care is available to every individual and family in every community. 3. Train primary care teams where people live and work. 4. Design information technology that serves the patient, family, and inter-professional care team."

If primary care can achieve all these objectives, then it would be transformational. It would deliver care that is COMPREHENSIVE, INTEGRATIVE, LONGITUDINAL, and PREVENTIVE.

Let us define each of those elements:

1. COMPREHENSIVE: Delivering and/or managing all elements of healthcare, e.g. this would include home healthcare at one end and specialty healthcare at the other.

2. INTEGRATIVE: Take a whole-patient-centered view and integrate all types of care, e.g. primary care should be aware of and take the lead in ensuring that all care that is delivered is coherent, e.g. the cardiologist does not prescribe medicine that the nephrologist treating the same patient feels could endanger kidney health.

3. LONGITUDINAL: The primary care physician should take responsibility for the healthcare journey of every patient from birth to death.

4. PREVENTIVE: Opportunities to prevent disease and interrupt the trajectory of lifestyle disease should be actively sought and taken advantage of. For example, the primary carer should provide weight and diet management, smoking cessation management, screening, counseling, risk identification, and risk mitigation interventions.

The new version of primary healthcare deserves a new name

Let us enumerate some of the characteristics of a primary care system that can strengthen Universal Health Coverage.

Primary healthcare as the backbone of Universal Health Coverage: A key enabling feature for primary care within Universal Healthcare is not only to act as the advocate for patient needs but also as the gatekeeper, ensuring that specialty care is provided when appropriate. Primary healthcare is not only the custodian of the needs of the patient but also the custodian of the processes that ensure that appropriate care is delivered at all times—neither too much care nor too little.

In such a system, every family will have a designated primary care contact person who will be familiar with the clinical histories of the citizen-users for whom they are accountable and can, therefore, triage the service needs appropriately. All elective consultations for care will flow through this designated point of contact.

Primary care must be available at the doorstep: Primary care must have the capacity to reach the homes of citizens. This feature will ensure that care is preventive; anticipating health conditions before they become critical and opening up opportunities to intervene early and pre-empt disease (e.g. weight reduction as a means to delay or prevent diabetes). We describe later in this section how technology-enabled community health workers can be deployed at scale at the front lines of healthcare, delivering to the homes of citizens preventive and even simple curative interventions.

Primary care should not become emergency care: Emergency care must be served by specialized healthcare centers that are equipped to manage a wide variety of emergencies. The outreach function of primary care through the community health worker can play a supportive role in providing first responder and resuscitative care, including the stabilization of vital parameters during the period before a patient reaches a specialized emergency healthcare center. This should be one of the tasks of the community health worker.

This new vision for primary care deserves a name change. We will call this model **Comprehensive Care** to distinguish it from the existing model. Correspondingly, the physician who delivers this will be the **Comprehensive Care Physician** (CCP).

360-degree care integration

In Comprehensive Care, the CCP (Comprehensive Care Physician) has a horizontal span (that includes pediatrics, obstetrics-gynecology, and geriatrics) similar to the current role for primary care physicians.

Comprehensive care is also vertically integrated: forward into the patient's home and backward to specialist secondary and tertiary care. It makes intuitive sense that the doctor who cares for the whole patient should also be responsible for coordinating care across every specialty that the patient encounters. Coordinating does not mean replacing the specialist's authority but ensuring that each specialty caring for the patient executes actions that are coordinated with the other specialists caring for the same patient.

Referrals to secondary care specialist doctors may be required at the start of treatment and episodically when a problem arises that the CCP is not equipped or trained to handle. Otherwise, routine follow-up care, monitoring, and adjustment of medications have to be done by the CCP. Graduating medical doctors may not have the depth of knowledge and skills to handle this increase in the span of their responsibilities, since medicine has become more sophisticated and nuanced in terms of diagnostics and therapeutics. Therefore, we envisage extensive deployment of care guidelines and treatment protocols, as well as extra training for graduate doctors given at regular intervals to keep them up to date. Finally, the CCP must have convenient access to specialist support via tele-health.

Gatekeeper function for Comprehensive Care

The Comprehensive Care Physician will be assigned a certain fixed population of families. For each family, there will be a designated CCP enabling a long-term temporal relationship between the CCP and the family. The CCP will also serve as a gatekeeper for secondary and tertiary care. Comprehensive Care will be the funnel through which all services are offered to the patient, thus forcing integration, both functional and temporal. This gatekeeper function will ensure that referrals for specialist care are kept to the appropriate minimum. Furthermore, when a patient has been to a tertiary care facility, she will be referred back to her CCP for follow-up care. The CCP will be the trusted owner of a patient's entire medical data and history including special health needs and information gathered during interactions with medical specialists and other health workers like physiotherapists.

In order to be an effective gatekeeper, care under UHC has to mandate that except in an emergency, the CCP has to be the first port of call for all medical needs. Mandates do not work unless they are coupled with incentives. The incentive in this case has to be that primary care delivered by the CCP and her team is completely free. There can be some form of non-financial accounting for the use of the system that credits the health account of each citizen a fixed number of healthcare credits each year that are used up every time a visit is undertaken to the CCP. Many clever variations of such a system can be designed so that there is a disincentive to overuse the system for trivial complaints while at the same time incentivizing behaviors such as annual health checks. The system can also be designed to incentivize physicians to prevent morbidity and improve the general health of the community.

The system envisaged above will not work unless we upgrade what CCPs can deliver. They must have a broader set of capabilities and expertise compared to what they are equipped with in the current system of training. Each CCP will have a number of Community Health Workers, as well as other medical staff whose work they supervise; they must have the ability to manage the team that they work with. On the other side, they must know how to understand and respond appropriately to treatment decisions guided by specialists.

Comprehensive care should be accountable to the local Community.

Comprehensive Care should be integrated with the community in multiple ways. For one, it should be accountable to local community leaders for its performance. The "Rogi Kalyan Samities (RKS)" as constituted under the National Health Mission (NHM) is an excellent construct in theory, but like many such initiatives, it falls short in practice. Accountability cannot be demanded unless the "Samities" are also well-informed to ask the right questions and demand performance against indicators that are clearly delineated and well-understood. Apart from this, how can we strengthen local governance of healthcare through structures like RKS? The NHM document already mentions the use of health NGOs to support the RKS. However, local ownership and drive can only come from local participants who are well-informed. The information gap can be filled by Community Health Workers who are recruited from the local population. Such CHWs can work with the RKS in an advisory capacity to help them understand the metrics that are designed to measure the health of the community in aggregate while also measuring individual patient experiences in using the system.

Healthcare is first and foremost a people business.

Healthcare is primarily a service industry, and therefore the people who man various positions are important if we are to deliver high-quality healthcare. Unlike most other service industry professionals, the healthcare worker is expected to demonstrate a high level of empathy for the patient. This fact has been recognized ever since we had family doctors in the 1800s. What has changed is the nature of medical practice. It has become highly fragmented, with each specialty drawing a moat around itself. While this can help train and develop specialists who become superb at a limited set of tasks, it is not a situation that is responsive to the needs of the whole patient. The lack of ownership for the outcomes for the whole patient also translates into a lack of empathy for the various needs of the patient beyond the immediate clinical episode.

The trend toward hyper-specialization in medical practice has also catapulted specialists to the top of the hierarchy. As specialists learn more and more about a smaller and smaller part of the patient, they get to earn more and more for doing less and less (e.g., we have interventional cardiologists who make a living mostly doing angioplasty). While hyperspecialism is an inevitable trend that is required in order to create focused experts who do work of high quality and efficiency, we must recognize that this does not serve the healthcare journey of the whole patient well. Therefore, we need organizational structures and work processes that drive authority and responsibility to the parts of healthcare that are not only the first to come directly in contact with the patient but also best placed to take responsibility for the whole patient—this is the Comprehensive Care Physician and her team.

In addition, the Comprehensive Care Physician will act as a patient advocate to compensate for the information asymmetry that exists in conversations between patients and the specialists who care for them. This specialist-facing role of the Comprehensive Care Physician complements her patient-facing role, i.e., being the first point of care for the patient and determining when a specialist referral is needed.

03 | HEALTHCARE IS BEST DELIVERED BY TEAMS

There are not enough primary care physicians in the country to fill all positions. Even in the current model of primary care, some 7.69% of PHCs do not have even a single doctor[9]. Given this shortage, the kind of personalized care we envision here cannot be delivered by doctors alone. Also, it is overkill to have highly trained physicians attend to issues like monitoring blood pressure, and adjusting medication for chronic conditions (things that can be protocol-driven and automated, with only exceptions being seen by the physician).

Teams should be the smallest indivisible units of healthcare service delivery

In the model of team-based care we propose, each physician should have under her supervision 15-20 health workers (Community Health Workers) along with whom she will constitute the healthcare team. The Community Health Worker (CHW) should be the absolute first point of contact for patients, except in an emergency. The CHW will be trained to perform 75% of the tasks the doctor would do, including things like physical examination and point of care diagnostics. Tele-health technology can tether each CHW to a Comprehensive Care Physician (CCP) for consultation and referral when needed. Each CCP and the tethered CHWs will constitute a team responsible for a certain number of families; say 5000 families (roughly, 20,000 individuals). In such a model, the CCP is elevated to take on more expertise-driven supervisory responsibilities. The role becomes attractive and aspirational for doctors, in keeping with the decade or more of training they undertake.

In this model the Comprehensive Care Physician (CCP) should handle and close more than 90% of consults without specialist referral. However, the CCP should have access to secondary care resources, including specialist colleagues who may even be co-located along with the CCP in the Comprehensive Care Center. Specialist physicians can be a readily available resource for the CCP through tele-health. A system of rotation where specialists spend a part of their time in the Comprehensive Care Center while retaining clinical responsibilities at a nearby hospital can be devised for situations where an in-presence consult is needed.

Team-based care is now the norm in every piece of healthcare, especially in hospitals. As clinical procedures become more complex, there is a need for additional experts and technicians to take responsibility for specialized pieces of care delivery, e.g. in cell therapy or organ transplantation. In team-based care, it is hard to place a greater or lesser value on the component pieces of care, since each piece contributes to the outcome. Teams, where the team members respect each other and work collaboratively, are key to success. Hierarchical models where a specialist at the top commands gofers at the bottom will not work.

A team-based approach to healthcare means that the center of authority in managing and coordinating the team must shift from its traditional locus toward other skilled workers who are not at the top of the traditional hierarchy in healthcare. Such coordinators must know how to assemble information and transmit synthesized information in an intelligible way so that the different specialists caring for a patient can make appropriate decisions. This role could be performed by a general physician or even a nurse on the team. In hospitals in the US, the "hospitalist" performs this role. For extremely sick patients suffering from diseases of multiple organs, the role of the "hospitalist" can be key in ensuring better outcomes. The role the "hospitalist" plays in care coordination in a hospital complements the role we envisage for the Comprehensive Care Physician at the front lines of care. We could, therefore, refer to the Comprehensive Care Physician as the "Comprehensivist" just as the generalist coordinator in the hospital is referred to as the "Hospitalist".

The shortage of doctors (and our inability to train them fast enough) at a time of expanding needs means that we have no option other than to expand the non-physician healthcare workforce exponentially and shift all routine procedures from physicians to this cadre. Experience has shown that task shifting of this kind improves the quality of care. This is explained by the fact that a trained non-physician health worker can spend more than the two minutes an average doctor consultation lasts in India, and therefore she can do a more thorough job than what the doctor can do.

Experience in the field has shown that health workers put through short training programs, with access to help from physicians via tele-health and ongoing training, can deliver high-quality care[10,11]. Such a workforce can be expanded significantly within a few years. This would also employ millions of young people. Such workers will get better with experience and can over time and with experience be shifted to tasks with increasing levels of complexity, e.g., managing emergencies in remote regions.

Technology is the glue that binds a team

Within the ecosystem, there exists a complex family of solutions that interdigitate with each other and are coordinated via a backbone of strong comprehensive (primary) healthcare. A corollary of this vision is the necessity for healthcare to be delivered at various points by individuals with varying skill sets. Each touchpoint has to come together with other touchpoints to form a whole that is not confusing for the patient. This is where the Electronic Health Record (EHR) can play a role. The EHR shared by all team members, from the Community Health Worker to the specialist in the hospital, can put all team members on the same page with respect to the care of a particular patient. The EHR becomes the glue that binds the team together.

The shared EHR is already in use to keep the entire teams on the same page during the care of a patient. Such sharing of information has the positive side effect of leveling hierarchies among team members, since it destroys traditional information silos that were used as levers of control by those privileged by their position to have access to information.

New roles in healthcare

New roles for healthcare workers will emerge as part of UHC. Healthcare workers, especially physicians, will be involved in the design and refinement of the processes that tie together the various components of healthcare. Managerial and leadership roles will require training a cadre specifically to perform such roles. These roles can be taken up by a dedicated cadre of MD-MBAs or Nurse-MBAs, thus ensuring that there is a good match between aptitude and the requirements of the job.

Healthcare workers will also be needed in building the public health infrastructure, from policymaking to design and implementation. These are higher-level tasks where the best generalist minds must engage. Such a structure, by default, puts Comprehensive Care and the Comprehensive Care Team as the central hub of healthcare, which is the appropriate place for them, since they have the big picture and the widest span of responsibility. This will also make roles in Comprehensive Care Teams coveted positions for which the best talent will vie.

We have outlined what a re-imagined Comprehensive Care System that delivers primary care should look like. In the essays that follow, we introduce the topic of the Hospital. We discuss to how we can reimagine the hospital by introducing focused care hospitals as a means to standardize care and thus achieve higher quality while lowering the cost of care. We also flesh out the details of the role of the front-line Community Health Worker.

04 | THE HOSPITAL

Aneurin Bevan, the Labor politician who was the architect of the NHS, is quoted as calling hospitals the "vertebrae of the health system". But this view has changed dramatically - recently, The Economist (27 May 2023) has called hospitals the "sponges" of healthcare for their proneness to sucking up all the money spent on healthcare. In the UK, hospitals consumed 65% of healthcare spending in 2018-19. Primary and community healthcare, only 19%.

If primary healthcare is so critical, why do we write at length about Hospitals? This is for the following reasons. Disease mitigation for non-communicable diseases is not foolproof; many of us will eventually become sick enough that we need interventional and curative care in a hospital setting. About 50% of lifetime healthcare costs are expended on hospital-based treatment—which is excessive, but that is the situation now. Over the next decade, DALYs due to non-communicable diseases are expected to go up by 20%, which will drive up hospitalization rates even more. Hospitalization is already expensive and is expected to become even more expensive in the future, as increasingly sophisticated medical interventions are put into play—organ replacement and cellular therapies, for example. Costly life-saving treatments can bankrupt individuals and even whole economies. Therefore, deliberate pre-emptive measures are warranted to make sure that these procedures are appropriately utilized and affordably priced. A great deal of attention will be needed to develop models that can bring down costs and improve efficiency. Hospitals are expensive and time-consuming to build— they are the oil tankers of healthcare, and therefore, budgeting for and designing new hospitals must be thought through very carefully, or else we will be sinking huge amounts in potential white elephants. Finally, hospitals are some of the most complex consumer-facing systems in modern societies, and they are becoming even more complex with advancements in medicine. This means that a combination of innovation, design thinking, and process re-engineering will be needed to ensure we can extract the highest possible productivity from hospitals. This will require research, analysis, leadership, and managerial skills of the highest order. It will also require politicians and policymakers to negotiate the delicate balance between competing priorities. They need to be prepared for this and not reflexively apply known facts to new problems. If the stakeholders can come together and get hospitals right, they can succeed against any challenge that the future holds. Building efficient hospitals is no less than "rocket science."

The prevailing model is a dinosaur

The prevailing model of the large multi-specialty general hospital is a dinosaur. Such hospitals are unable to keep up with the demands of a rapidly evolving healthcare environment: they do not generate surpluses of a magnitude to satisfy owners, they do not provide work environments that satisfy doctors, and most importantly, they do not consistently satisfy patients. This may be dismissed simply as part of the general malaise afflicting healthcare. We argue, however, that while hospitals do suffer the difficulties that afflict healthcare in general, they also suffer from a unique set of problems. And unless we fix these issues, we cannot fix healthcare. The tsunami of technology and social change coming at us will put existing hospitals under extreme stress, endangering their ability to provide quality care at a reasonable cost.

Why not let things evolve organically as the marketplace grows and evolves? Simple market forces can, in the short term, valorize the needs of the dominant players of the day; currently, most investment in hospital capacity is by the private sector. Allowing private capital to distort the demand-supply equations in healthcare can be disastrous for evolving any kind of equitable and affordable hospital system. This is one sector where the Government has to take a direct coordinating and regulating role. Experts in the government, the medical sector, and healthcare policy must develop appropriate models for the evolution of hospitals. We do not need a centrally regulated command and control hospital economy. But the government must play the role of a market maker: ensuring fairness, a level playing field for all comers, including start-ups, and providing strategic support (financial and infrastructural) where required.

The multi-specialty hospital tries to be the Swiss knife of healthcare

Hospitals come in many sizes and flavors. Everything from the massive 5000-plus-bed hospital coming up in Patna to the 10-bed nursing home in your neighborhood is called a hospital. For this discussion, we are focusing on the larger, 100-plus-bed multi-specialty hospitals, although the comments may apply equally to hospitals of all sizes and types.

The multi-specialty hospital is like a Swiss knife. It tries to do everything for everyone. What does this mean? It will provide everything from treatment for an ingrown toenail to a heart transplant. It will do everything from simple outpatient consultations for diabetes to complex robotic surgery.

Some hospitals can favorably be compared to 7-star hotels in terms of the creature comforts they provide. Such hospitals cater to the ultra-rich—people who occupy a rarefied slice of the economy where the depths of their pockets determine what is delivered as part of the packaged experience. In this book, we are not focusing on such institutions. We concern ourselves mainly with essential healthcare that every citizen needs as part of their requirement for basic health. Hence, we focus on the bread-and-butter government hospitals and not-for-profit hospitals, as well as corporate hospitals that provide advanced first-world treatments in a modest cost-friendly ambience.

Since this book is all about how hospitals need to evolve in response to a changing environment, it may help to start by recounting a fairly typical hospitalization experience. Hospitals are frequently criticized when citizens talk about their healthcare experience. This recounting is meant to be representative of the many unsatisfactory encounters we have with our healthcare delivery systems.

A Hospitalization Experience

Thankfully, we see the insides of hospitals more often as solicitous visitors than as patients. If you require hospitalization, your illness is likely to be something serious. The view of the hospital from the bedside is vastly different from the view of the hospital from the bed. When you are in bed, you are not in control of your fate, and you are not in a position to dictate choices. The word "Hospitalization" refers to something done to you and not something you do for yourself. It is no wonder, for most of us, it is an unpleasant memory. In a chapter on Hospitals - where they are and where they are going - it is worthwhile to start by recounting the experience of a patient who had to undergo the ordeal of hospitalization. The following description is of a specific patient's experience (one of us), but the script follows a pattern that most have-been patients will recognize.

One fine morning, you wake up feeling sick enough that you feel that you need to quickly get to a hospital. You have a friend who happens to work in one of the corporate multi-specialty hospitals nearby, and so that is where you head. You enter a cavernous space where many other unfortunate people wait (patiently, what else!). If you are lucky, you enter on your own feet, retaining a semblance of agency for a short period before you lose it along with any pretense you had of being a person. Depending on the urgency of your situation (and, in my case, my influence with the doctor on duty), the wait for the next step to happen can vary from as little as five minutes to several hours. You are then ushered into the presence of a brusquely efficient person in a white coat, usually in a much smaller, low-ceilinged room in a recess in the hospital. It bears a resemblance to the inner sanctum sanctorum in a temple. The person in the white coat — the doctor — is priestly in his demeanor. His admonitions and prescriptions are like incantations, delivered with suitable gravitas. He sizes up your "monetizability" by asking some questions about your profession, where you work, etc., and then passes you on for further processing. You are rolled around by the attendant pushing your wheelchair, and the paperwork is done for you. The admission process is generally swift if your ability to pay is in no doubt in the eyes of the admission clerk; if you fail the money test, you can still get through by delivering a lump of cash upfront. The urgency to bed you is not matched by an urgency to start treatment. Instead, you are subjected to an interminable litany of testing; some of the tests are to the point and relevant to your complaints, for others, there seems to be no purpose except to use up idle diagnostic capacity in the hospital. By this time, there is a heaviness in your heart that seems to grow in proportion with the accumulating charges. And then the moment comes. The pronouncement of the verdict at your bedside. Unfortunately, the verdict is vague, signaling that all the testing and prodding (these days there is vastly more testing and almost no prodding) have been of no help in pinning down the diagnosis. A further round of testing ensues, including the insertion of tubes into your body and the placement of the body inside a tube. This additional round of scanning is inconclusive (although the scamming that underpins it is very productive for the hospital owners). Fortunately, by this time you are feeling better and are pronounced fit enough to go home, but not before you are offered a laparoscopic procedure to remove some innocent stones in your gall bladder that were picked up on some of the images. You refuse to be bullied into a procedure which, according to you, is like treating the bystanders when there is a road accident; you would rather leave those innocent stones alone. The doctor through carefully chosen phrases leaves you with the feeling that you are making a huge mistake, for which you will no doubt end up paying a big price down the road.

It is time for the big day when you finally feel whole again after having been treated as an assembly of organs. You are given permission to go home. You feel stronger and in control. You are ready to return home ASAP. Except for one last cloud in the silver lining - after several ping-pong conversations with the insurance agent, you discover that your policy is not as "cashless" as promised, and you are unshackled and allowed to leave the premises only after you have unloaded some more cash. You are handed an unintelligible discharge summary, which is so mistaken in its premise that it may well belong to another patient. The line items in the bill are in obscure and unchallengeable code. In any case, you are so desperate to reach home that you are in no mood to engage over the minutiae of the bill. You are fondly asked to return after a month for some further prodding and poking, with no assurance that the second round of prodding and poking will unmask anything more germane than the vague findings from the first round. It will, however, further lighten the weight of your purse and give employment to several already well-fed medical professionals.

The above Kafkaesque experience of hospitalization is personal - one of us went through this. If you, the reader, have ever had to experience hospitalization in one of our swanky hospitals, you may be reading this with a sense of déjà vu. Most patients who visit hospitals come away with mixed feelings about the experience - joy if the illness is healed, commingled with frustration at the unsatisfactoriness of everything else relating to the whole event. You promise yourself never to become sick enough to be at the receiving end of a hospitalization.

Despite all the negativism about hospitals, we cannot wish away their existence. They still are the most powerful means to deliver curative care. But this was not always the case. For much of their existence, hospitals were less about cure and more about prayer to ensure a place in heaven when you die; a fate more commonplace when prayer was the only tool in the hands of the priest who doubled as a doctor. The inflexion point at which hospitals changed from their original avatar as prayerful places where the soul was healed to today's technopolises that focus exclusively on the body is bracketed by two paintings in the city of Philadelphia. Let us take a small excursion and view those paintings and what they tell us about the dramatic discontinuity hospitals experienced in the late 19th century.

The origin of hospitals: The Eakins Paintings

Although institutions resembling the modern hospital have been around since medieval times, the modern hospital evolved largely in the post-war era in the 20th century. The seeds of the hospital, as we know it today, were laid in the 19th century. Two paintings by the Philadelphian Thomas Eakins bookend 15 years in the late 19th Century when developments in antisepsis, nursing, and anesthesia made surgery the safe, painless, and effective procedure that it is today.

The first painting, titled 'The Gross Clinic,' was executed in 1875 in time for its display at the US Centennial Expo—a showcase of advances in American Technology and Science in the hundred years since independence. Eakins, a student of anatomy, chose Samuel D. Gross, a famous Philadelphia surgeon who practiced at the Jefferson Medical College, as the protagonist for the scene he depicted. Painted vertically on a canvas 8 feet tall and 6 feet wide, it captures a moment during a surgical procedure when Gross turns away from the patient on the operating table to face the students in the observation gallery around him. His face, turned in the direction of the person viewing the painting, is lit up by a ray of light that shines directly on his head from above him, perhaps from a skylight; it was a time before artificial lighting was available, and surgeries were scheduled midday to take advantage of natural lighting. Gross stands tall and imperious. His posture is godlike, especially in comparison to the small figure of an old woman behind him who is shielding her face from the gory sight in front of her. She seems to be the mother of the boy who is being operated upon, as he lies held doubled over on a wooden trestle table, his thigh exposed for surgery. The incision wound is open and retracted. Gross's hand grips the scalpel, from which blood is still dripping, even as his distant gaze appears to remove him from any concern for the patient on the table. What is most remarkable about the scene from today's perspective is the complete absence of any sterile precautions. Gross is still in his street clothes, as are his assistants. The surgical instruments are laid out in a tray in the foreground, with no indication that they have been sterilized for surgery. An assistant holds down the boy's legs as another assistant continues the surgical procedure from which Gross has been momentarily diverted. This realistic depiction of a barbaric procedure being carried out in primitive conditions created such a public outcry that the painting was consigned to a less visited corner of the expo.

Fourteen years later, in 1889, Thomas Eakins was commissioned by students at the University of Pennsylvania to create a painting of a famous surgeon at the university, D. Hayes Agnew. The changes that Eakins captures in comparison to the earlier painting are remarkable. Agnew is less godlike, and he is portrayed with more human proportions. The theater is well-lit under artificial light, and the students in the gallery are clearly visible. The patient is a woman, and her face is visible, giving her the humanity that was missing from the patient in the previous painting. Agnew and his assistants are in surgical gowns and white coats. The operating table seems to have been designed for the purpose and is appropriately draped to maintain a sterile surgical field. The surgical instruments are kept in a tray filled with fluid, probably carbolic acid, to keep them sterile. There is also an additional presence in the room—a nurse in uniform. She stands calm and impassive as she oversees the surgery, ready to hand instruments to the surgeons. The Agnew Clinic, in its portrayal of surgery with proper sterile precautions and absence of gore, may have been intended as a commentary on the changes the artist had seen in surgical practice in that short period. Antisepsis alone brought down the death rate from surgery by 99%. Anesthesia gave surgeons enough time to perform complex surgery without worrying about the patient waking up.

These developments would remove the last constraints to using surgery, even as a pre-emptive measure, to cure disease. With the growth of surgery, the need for hospitals where patients could be kept for prolonged post-surgical observation periods grew.

The next inflection point for the development of hospitals came as a result of advances in biomedicine, specifically the mass production of penicillin. Interestingly, the discovery of penicillin by Alexander Fleming also took place in a hospital—St. Mary's in London. Once penicillin became available for use in the early 1940s, infections that were once considered fatal became treatable. All kinds of bacterial infections: meningitis, pneumonia, and endocarditis, could now be effectively treated in a hospital using penicillin. Surgical wound infections could be cured, and clinical outcomes for surgery improved considerably, permitting surgeons to enhance the scope of surgery. Many surgical innovations took place in the battlefields of the two world wars.

The modern multi-specialty hospital

Today's large multi-specialty hospitals with thousands of beds are the behemoths of healthcare. The primitive medieval structures were first replaced by pavilion-style structures that were spacious, well-lit, and cross-ventilated. Today's hospitals use space more efficiently - they are large multi-story complexes that co-locate all the modern technologies on offer. Whether it is the operating room or a patient room, the kind of equipment that goes into them can seem straight out of a Sci-Fi film (Da Vinci robots, proton beams, cyclotrons).

The biggest hospitals in India are all in the Government sector, with the largest being Ahmedabad Civil Hospital with over 4000 beds. The largest in the private sector is Medanta Medicity with 1500 beds. Patna Medical College Hospital in Bihar will become the largest hospital in the world (the incumbent with that title is the West China Medical Center of Sichuan University with 4300 beds) when the redevelopment project with 5462 beds is completed. Bigger seems to be better when it comes to hospitals. We will see in later sections whether this aspiration to be the biggest is justified given the changing trends in hospitals.

A 100-bed hospital can require more than 100,000 square feet of space (at approximately 1000 square feet per patient in a bed). Many of the first corporate hospitals were built expansively and lavishly in a fit of untempered hubris. As much as 1200 square feet per patient bed was the norm. Since then, on a per-bed basis, hospitals have shrunk, and outstanding hospitals are designed with space allocation of 600 to 800 square feet per patient bed. A part of this shrinkage comes from the smaller footprint of new-age imaging technologies, which is perhaps compensated on the upside by the proliferation of new, alternative imaging technologies. Since hospitals have to be in central urban locations where access is easy, preferably near hotels, public transportation, etc., they occupy the most expensive real estate in the city. A 100-bed hospital can require 3–4 acres of prime land in the central business district.

Large hospitals that house multiple specialties, each specialty with its complement of gleaming new equipment, have been described by Clayton Christensen as examples of the 'solution shop model' (we used this term in the context of primary healthcare earlier in this section). There is nothing they cannot do. All kinds of problems can be thrown at them, and they will apply their formidable technologies to find a solution. In short, they are designed to solve unstructured problems.

The layers of organizational complexity needed for this 'solution shop model' may appear like neat layers of a crème cake. But this is deceptive. The complexity is enervating to the operations of the hospital. Every time an additional layer of complexity is added, more things can and do go wrong. Public health researcher Ashish Jha calls US hospitals the most dangerous place for Americans: 15-20% of patients going to a hospital suffer serious consequences of medical error. This applies even more to private for-profit hospitals, where profit is often prioritized over safety.

Hospitals Redux

From their pre-eminent position, hospitals lost some of their cachet as ultimate providers in the 1990s. Several developments triggered this change. One was the trend of early mobilization after surgery. While the traditional perception of post-operative recovery was that it was a time when the body healed and, therefore, needed to be taken at a slow pace, it increasingly became clear that long immobilization post-surgery was bad for clinical outcomes. The Swiss AO group (an Association of Surgeons Specialized in treating skiing injuries and fractures) experimented with early mobilization of fracture patients by using plates and screws to instantaneously stabilize the fractured bone. Following this, other specialties like cardiac surgery also experimented with quick mobilization and found that results were improved when post-operative bed rest time was reduced. In the 1980s, it was common for patients to spend a week or more in the hospital after a coronary artery bypass graft. Now, if you have a stent placed in a coronary vessel, you could be home the very next day. If you needed open-heart surgery, it could be a few days more and mostly in intensive care, but it is rarely a full week in the hospital before discharge. Some studies show that patients who are discharged the same day after joint replacement surgery fare as well as patients kept in the hospital for several days. Clinical outcomes improve with shorter hospital stays.

Apart from technologies like keyhole and laparoscopic surgery that reduce the trauma of surgery, there were several other drivers for reducing hospitalization. These were - the need to reduce costs, the need to spread the utilization of expensive hospital equipment over a larger number of patients, the fear of hospital-acquired infections with longer stays, and patient preference. For some diseases, e.g. duodenal ulcers, new drugs like histamine receptor antagonists and proton pump inhibitors proved so effective that surgery, in most cases, became unnecessary. More recently, the rise of the home care industry has made possible sophisticated home care, including the possibility of replicating many aspects of an ICU in the patient's home. Companies like Portea provide a nurse, a hospital bed, home visits by doctors, and all the monitoring equipment required for care at home, including perfusion lines. This of course, comes at a high price. Broadly, these trends are resulting in a net reduction in the demand for hospital beds.

If the above comments portray a picture of the hospital as declining in importance, then this view is only one side of the coin. The area where hospitals excel is acute intensive care, hospitals with their team-based approach to the acutely sick patient deliver care that cannot be easily replicated outside the large hospital support structure. Correspondingly, while regular hospital beds decline in numbers, the US has seen an increase in acute care beds. The aging of the population and increases in chronic illness with multi-organ involvement, the requirement for sophisticated invasive multi-parameter monitoring, and the need for tightly managed and rapid responses to patient conditions are also increasing the need for acute care beds. Treatments are also becoming more sophisticated: organ replacement, prostheses, cell-based treatments, gene therapy, extracorporeal membrane oxygenation (ECMO), Intra-aortic Balloon Pumps (IABP), hemodialysis, and treatments that use robots or radioisotopes. The hospital is being reincarnated in a new avatar, as a place where medical marvels are enabled through a combination of scientific medicine and technology. Some of these marvels are so expensive to deploy that only a large regional hospital can afford to build them in the first place.

The impending transformation of the Hospital

Hospitals are a strange blend of traditions carried over from 100 years ago alongside modern curative technologies. Hospitals must change so that they can deliver on the potential benefits of the new technologies. The changes that are needed take many forms - some transformational and some incremental. Shorter time in bed in the hospital means that turnover rates for hospital beds are high. Higher turnover rates make hospitals, with their costly infrastructure and highly paid staff, economically viable.

Hospitals will increasingly specialize by organ (e.g., a kidney or eye hospital) or a subset of elective procedures (e.g., joint replacement or organ transplantation or cell and gene therapy) since it does not work very well to mix "solution shop" style services with services that are more effectively delivered using a "factory" model (more on this later). Hospitals will also be more compact and modular, allowing for flexibility in space utilization. Acute care and long-term care will be segregated. There will be new mini-hospitals that are located within the community where the patient lives.

The Comprehensive Care Physician and her hospital counterpart, the Hospitalist, will ensure coordination between different pieces of the ecosystem. Large hospitals will be embedded in this ecosystem and networked with other players. Patients will be empowered with data and advice throughout the care process and will participate as informed equals in the clinical decision-making process. New specialisms will emerge, customized to the needs of patients in a hospital environment. Hospital care has traditionally been fractured across the many disciplines that serve severely sick patients. Hospitalists bridge disciplines and help deliver coordinated care in a hospital environment, similar to what a Comprehensive Care Physician does at the front line of care. Even more important will be the emergence of new auxiliary roles - technicians who will perform many of the procedures physicians perform today, e.g., closing surgical wounds, complex catheterization and placement of indwelling cannulas.

Acute care facilities will operate in a truly 24/7 fashion, with extra effort taken to ensure that there is no difference in the quality of care at night or daytime or between weekdays and weekends. Specialists will work shifts so that staffing quality is the same at all times of the day. From the biomedical model of health, where Organ Replacement has become standard practice, we are moving toward the Molecular Model of Health where Genetic Engineering has allowed precision crafting of cell behaviors that enable the repair of disease at the molecular level. The pace at which these changes will happen will depend on the socioeconomic and political context within which healthcare is placed.

In all this, there will be recognition that hospitals cannot be everything to everyone. Hospitals will learn to specialize and also dial down their offerings based on what society can afford. We have to recognize the reality that resources are not infinite, and care has to be rationed. But this rationing should be planned and based on concepts of equity and not on economic relativism of the kind that places different values on lives purely based on things like earning potential. At the same time, the system has to allow the wealthy to buy the care they demand. If a rich actor needs liposuction or a facelift, they should be in a position to buy such care at whatever price it is available. But essential care should be available to all citizens, whether they can pay for it or not. In the coming chapters, we will explore all these issues and more.

As a part of the solution for the ills that plague the multi-specialty hospital model, we have also devoted space for a separate discussion of hospitals designed as focused factories—a design already in place and working effectively in specialties like eye care and orthopedics. But these historical implementations have been reactive—a response engendered by the specialty in which the founder of the hospital is qualified. We see focused factories as a proactive "design" response that can deliver quality healthcare, both economically and at scale.

Furthermore, we could not leave untouched an unfortunate tendency among planners and policymakers to create clones of AIIMS (All India Institute of Medical Science, New Delhi) as a bridge to fill gaps in healthcare. They are inadvertently creating behemoths that will gobble an increasing share of resources to deliver costly care inefficiently. The difficulty in finding specialist doctors to staff these new AIIMS and the inherent complexity of the multi-specialty general hospital model will result in a slide in the quality of care at these new institutions.

Too many AIIMS will simply make us sicker

The Government has recently announced the creation of 25 All India Institutes of Medical Sciences (AIIMS), of which 15 have already been built. This is a lazy supply-driven response. If building a better hospital in different parts of the country modeled on AIIMS in Delhi was the solution, then this initiative has meaning. Simply scaling up and replicating existing models cannot solve the problem when the context changes. We need to look closely at what is needed and try to customize our hospital systems to meet that specific need at the lowest possible cost without sacrificing the quality of care. The AIIMS model cannot achieve this objective. But can this be done? We believe it can. Elsewhere in this book, we provide analysis backed by empirical research to show a few models that can get us there. None of them calls for building more AIIMS-style institutions. Regardless, these changes cannot be brought about overnight. We expect the full-scale transformation of tertiary care delivery models (side by side with changes in other parts of the healthcare value chain) to take at least two decades. This also underpins the need to start working on this now and gradually shape the trajectory in a manner to intercept a desirable end state in the 2030s.

The All India Institute of Medical Science (AIIMS, Delhi) was established as a national institute of excellence, for medical research and for training doctors. A secondary expectation was that AIIMS-trained doctors would go to other parts of the country and seed the creation of new AIIMS-like centers of excellence in healthcare delivery. AIIMS has partly achieved the first objective: The institute's faculty publishes more research papers than their counterparts at peer institutions within India, although not as many high-quality papers as the best institutions in the world. The second aim was never met, since the elitist environment at AIIMS meant that they were unlikely to go anywhere else in India except to another elite institution or overseas. Instead of being a pipeline for qualified talent, AIIMS sequestered some of the best medical talent away from places where it was most needed.

AIIMS' reputation makes it a magnet for patients from outside Delhi: AIIMS sees more than 7,000 patients each day, of whom a large chunk come from the states surrounding Delhi. If AIIMS is such a magnet for patients, it makes good sense to set up more AIIMS-like institutions. This is the logic driving the establishment of 25 AIIMS clones across India. However, this may inhibit the progress of primary health care and district hospitals. Which patient would want to be treated at a district hospital when an AIIMS is a bus ride away? Which doctor would want to work in a district hospital that has neither equipment nor status when a job at an AIIMS can provide both?

When a foundation for basic public health care does not exist, then constructing a costly super-specialty tertiary health care facility will be a death blow to any attempt to push the agenda of public health. First, it will soak up resources (capital and personnel), leaving only leftovers for public health. Second, it will accelerate the race among private hospitals to build sophisticated and costly infrastructure to compete with the nearby AIIMS. The private hospitals will then use all means available to fill the capacity, leading to a ballooning of wasteful care and costs. Finally, plonking AIIMS all across India will act as a strong disincentive for local governments to build primary and secondary care infrastructure. Yet another unintended consequence of establishing these islands of excellence and plenty is that they will concentrate large numbers of patients within their premises, impairing the quality of service and increasing problems such as antibiotic resistance and iatrogenic morbidity.

It is not that we do not need AIIMS-like institutions. But we may only need four to six such institutions across the country. Like AIIMS, Delhi, they must be designed specifically to carry out advanced biomedical research and preferably operate as postgraduate institutions that focus on the introduction of cutting-edge methods in health care. Co-locating them with engineering and science research institutions such as the Indian Institutes of Technology and the Indian Institutes of Science can have a synergistic effect.

To deliver health care at scale without compromising quality, we need a different kind of hospital. First, we need our hospitals to be embedded in and seamlessly integrated within a network of healthcare providers from primary to tertiary care. A system of referrals should determine who needs to go to a tertiary care facility for treatment. Plain vanilla multi-specialty hospitals should give way to a mix of focused care facilities (e.g., hospitals that specialize in a single specialty, like cardiac care), emergency care facilities, and community hospitals (that can take on the workload of highly routine procedures). Only such a differentiated yet fully integrated healthcare network can provide high-quality care close to where the patients live, at a cost the national budget can bear.

For a big chunk of our population, quality healthcare is a luxury. Giving them access to a super-specialty hospital when their basic health needs are not met is like Marie Antoinette asking starving Parisians to eat cake. Instead of asking them to go to a distant AIIMS, the State should discharge its responsibility in providing them seamless end-to-end healthcare that starts close to their home at a primary health center.

Focused factories of healthcare

If a resource-constrained nation like India has to achieve the twin goals of affordable and quality health care for all, it will require drastic re-engineering of the healthcare delivery model. India faces two main realities: a large population and low per capita GDP, leaving little room for the substantial investments necessary to build healthcare infrastructure. An acute shortage of doctors outside major metropolitan areas further compounds the problem. The rapid growth in the prevalence of chronic non-communicable diseases threatens to transform a critical issue into one of apocalyptic dimensions. Successive governments have attempted to bridge the gap between supply and demand by applying band-aid fixes, for example, by opening more super-specialty hospitals. This is neither affordable when done at the required scale, nor an appropriate response to the supply-demand gap in healthcare.

While primary healthcare has to be the backbone on which any healthcare system is built, we should not be blind to the needs of vast numbers of Indians awaiting hospital-based tertiary care for illnesses like heart disease and cancer. Cardiac surgeon Devi Shetty (Narayana Health) has stated that a country of India's size requires 2.5 million heart surgeries to be performed each year. About 100,000 are performed on wealthy patients who can afford expensive private hospitals. The rest wait endlessly for their turn at overstretched government hospitals, and most die before they get the care they need. A recent article in the medical journal The Lancet estimates that close to 2.4 million Indians die each year due to lack of access to healthcare or poor-quality healthcare.

Problems with the General Hospital Model

The classic tertiary (hospital-based) healthcare facility is a General Hospital (GH), a multi-specialty facility that treats everyone and handles everything, from the most complex multimodal treatments to more straightforward procedures in specialized areas like dentistry, ophthalmology, and ENT. A majority of patients fall into the latter category, requiring the services of a single specialty using procedures that can be standardized. A multi-purpose GH, by trying to optimize resources and processes across multiple specialties, ends up being suboptimal for all.

The GH model brings under one roof the treatment of both complex and straightforward cases, conflating business models with incompatible metrics of output, value, and payment. This results in a needless increase in cost and impairment of quality.

The GH model is also highly capital-intensive. Given the need to cater to multiple specialties, these hospitals become bloated bureaucracies. They are doctor-centric and not patient-centric in their business processes. Furthermore, high fixed costs inflate the cost of treatment. Co-locating different specialties that have different needs makes it impossible to allocate costs of staffing and space accurately.

The complex organization of the GH and the inability to tightly link input costs to output value leads to undisciplined billing practices and ballooning hospital bills.

The hospital as a focused factory

The optimization problem General Hospitals face is similar to the optimization problem faced by the large unspecialized manufacturing organizations set up in the US in the 1960s and 1970s. Focused factories that specialize in a limited set of products were mooted as a response. In the 1990s, Harvard professor Regina Herzlinger put forward the idea of focused factories as a solution for the problems plaguing healthcare.

Focused Healthcare Factories (FHF) specialize in a limited set of specialties and clinical processes. The Georgia Sickle Cell Center in Atlanta is an example of an FHF that arose as a response to the poor outcomes achieved in sickle cell patients at non-specialized centers. In eight years, this one-stop-shop halved hospital admissions and cut emergency admissions by 80 percent. The Shouldice Hernia Hospital in Ontario specializes in hernia surgery. The cost of a hernia repair at Shouldice is 30 percent lower than the reimbursement rate in the US. This lower cost is achieved with better outcomes—a complication rate of 0.5 percent versus 5-10 percent outside. Similarly, the Coxa Hospital for Joint Replacement in Finland has a complication rate of 0.1 percent vs. a rate of 10-12 percent at a GH performing the same procedure. As a test, the cardiac surgery practice at the Mayo Clinic prospectively carved out a Focused Care Practice within its larger Solution Shop model practice and found that implementation of the model reduced resource use, length-of-stay, and cost. Variation was markedly reduced, and outcomes were improved.

FHFs work so well since they permit standardization of care using an algorithmic approach to clinical processes. Embedding repeatable and controllable processes along the whole sequence of patient care, from admission to discharge, allows such facilities to deliver predictable high-quality outcomes. The standardization enables tasks to be shifted down the clinical hierarchy to junior doctors and even nurses, thus lowering costs without compromising quality. FHF also enables steeper learning curves for staff due to the high volumes. The experience of the staff and the structured learning environment create conditions that are congenial for innovation and continuous improvement.

For FHFs to impact healthcare, the concept of the FHF has to be scaled up nationally. The for-profit sector may not be best suited to orchestrate this. The government must play its role and seed the creation of FHFs in partnership with healthcare NGOs and physician cooperatives. Since this will take time, the government could, as an intermediate step, carve out embedded FHFs within large government hospitals. Such units must be independently resourced and have sufficient autonomy in operation. Individual FHFs can become nodes in a nationally interconnected grid. Such a grid will enable smaller and remotely located FHFs to access the knowledge footprint of the virtual network. For example, standardized care protocols can be distributed from a central node, and purchasing cost efficiencies can be maximized by consolidating the requirements of the network when negotiating with vendors. The FHF model has already taken root in specialties: eye care and obstetrics. The National Cancer Grid is an example of how such a model can be deployed to serve the vast numbers of cancer patients across the country. The task now is to re-purpose this experience in other specialties.

India is uniquely placed to deliver high-quality, affordable healthcare to the masses. The FHF leverages India's enormous patient numbers to create a model that delivers scalable, high-quality care at a lower cost. If India can marry its skills in executing large-scale mission-oriented projects with its information technology capabilities, there is no reason why it cannot be a global epicenter for high-quality healthcare. Such capabilities will also be attractive to patients from other countries that do not have the critical mass required to build similar large-scale, high-volume healthcare networks.

Separating focused elective care from emergency care creates the best of all worlds. Focused care hospitals provide higher quality at lower costs. At the same time, since they are designed mainly to provide elective care, their distance from where patients live (accessibility) is not an issue. Emergency care hospitals that are compact, specialized, and freestanding can be made more accessible by having more of them distributed closer to the community. Their smaller footprint can lower costs while at the same time providing the convenience of rapid access when an emergency occurs. Emergency care hospitals are also, in a sense, focused care hospitals. Except that they are focused on providing purely "solution shop" style healthcare delivery for emergencies. Their focused approach to emergency care will also result in better clinical outcomes. This is an example of breaking the stranglehold of the iron triangle. Traditional zero-sum thinking must be replaced by more innovative thinking about alternate business models that can deliver on multiple axes at the same time. Indian hospitals like Aravind Eye Care have shown that this is possible in the context of Focused Care business models.

The focused care model cannot be universalized. We still need hospitals that operate as "solution shops," and we also need teaching hospitals where young doctors and other medical professionals can be trained in a broad range of disciplines. Therefore, the GH model of the hospital will have to coexist with focused healthcare facilities. There is also a need for what we term para-hospitals, i.e., hospitals that provide step-down care such as long-term post-acute care rehabilitation services. Especially for a country like India where socioeconomic realities make it difficult to provide such care at home, there is a need for such para-hospitals where the patients' family can participate in care-giving under the supervision of nurses in a hostel-like environment. This will enable the provision of such care at a lower cost to everyone needing it. Finally, while the Comprehensive Community Care Centers will have provision for minor surgeries, there is still a need for nursing homes in the community that can provide episodic care for chronic diseases, e.g. frequent hospital admissions for cardiac failure. So, while the FHF model will streamline and make more efficient the provision of certain standardized elective procedures, other specialized care delivery institutions will coexist.

How many beds for how many heads?

The default assumption is that India has fewer hospital beds than it requires since we spend less than other countries on healthcare. Based on this, there is a clamor to build more hospitals. If we need to plan for additional hospital bed capacity, we must start by asking ourselves - how many hospital beds does India already have? Unfortunately, there is no authenticated source for this information. While data about beds in government-owned hospitals seems reasonably accurate, estimates about the private sector are approximations! In its report released in Nov 2019 titled "Health System for a New India: Building Blocks," the NITI Aayog says - "the typical private hospital has just 20 to 30 beds, though an undetermined number are much smaller". These hospitals, frequently referred to as "nursing homes," also operate with fewer staff: one-third of private hospitals reported having only one worker in 2010-11, while just over two-thirds reported five or fewer workers. Consumption of in-patient services is driven by multiple factors. Apart from the severity of the medical condition, other factors, such as preferences of the treating doctor, payment options available (self-pay or insurance), and excess available bed capacity, all play a role in determining whether a patient is admitted for treatment. This can be illustrated with an example. The C-section or Cesarean section is the most common surgical procedure requiring hospital admission in India. As per current estimates, around 4 million C-Sections are performed in India every year. Assuming a 3-day stay per procedure, and 300 service days per hospital bed, we would require 40,000 beds, which works out to approximately three beds per 100,000 population. C-sections in government hospitals account for ~ 15% of all deliveries, whereas in private sector hospitals, C-sections account for more than 33% of all deliveries for patients paying out of pocket. The proportion of C-sections for patients with health insurance may be even higher at 60% of total deliveries. This excess use of

C-sections is driven by non-medical considerations, e.g. profitability of C-section over normal delivery. If the proportion of C-Sections is reduced to 15% of all deliveries, as recommended by the WHO, the total number of C-Sections performed would drop to 2.85 million, and the total beds required would then be only 28,000 per 100,000! The 15% cap should allow all medically necessary C-Sections to be carried out. Whimsical preferences driven by non-medical considerations can have a big effect on the consumption of hospital beds.

So, how many beds do we need? Tracking the utilization of existing hospital bed capacity can help us understand the demand for in-patient services. A caveat we must bear in mind is that all hospital beds are not the same. Even within the same hospital, a bed in the critical care area is vastly different from one in the general ward or one in a daycare unit. There will be differences in bed composition between hospitals in terms of space allocation, infrastructure, or staffing. The two key factors that influence this are: what kind of procedures they support and what disease prevalence in the local area they cater to. The pattern of utilization of hospital beds combined with epidemiological data as well as data on disease burden can provide insights into the reasons for hospitalization and the kind of procedures being performed. It is likely that, due to a variety of reasons, not all the demand for any particular procedure will get converted into addressable demand. Once again, let us look at childbirth, which is the top reason for hospitalization. Given the current India birth rate of ~18/1000, annual childbirth numbers are in the ballpark of 24 million. Of these, around 79% are institutional deliveries, which is lower compared to developed countries. For simplicity if we assume just two kinds of procedures, the normal delivery with a 2-day stay, and a C-Section with a 3-day stay, and that C-Sections account for 20% of the total, the calculation looks as follows:

Estimating bed requirement for childbirths				
S.No	Description	Nos	Units	Remarks/ explanations
1	Total childbirths per year	24	Mil	
2	Institutional childbirths per year	19	Mil	79% of all childbirths
3	Normal childbirths per year	15	Mil	~80% of institutional, 2 day stay
4	C-Sections	4	Mil	~20% of institutional, 3 day stay
5	Hospital Service Days/year	300	Days	
6	Therefore total Bed days required for childbirth	42	Mil Bed Days	(15 Mil*2 days) + (4 Mil*3 days)
7	Beds required for the above	140000	Beds	42 Mil Bed days/300 days

Any change in the base case assumptions can swing the numbers significantly. For instance, if the length of stay were to be 4 days for a C-Section, the total number of beds required could be ~ 153,000, which is almost 10% higher. So clearly, data flowing from the utilization of existing beds is crucial to forecast the incremental number of beds required. Utilization data can also reveal the occupancy rates of existing capacity. It is not unusual for longer duration stays (especially in a private sector hospital), not due to a medical necessity, but because spare capacity exists (supply-driven consumption of medical services; a kind of waste that is covered in the next section). Placing this alongside global benchmarks for appropriate care can also inform us about the right number of beds required to support the demand for procedures performed in an inpatient setting.

How much does a hospital bed cost?

It is not enough to know how many beds we need. We also need to estimate what the additional capacity will cost. When working out the cost per hospital bed, the costs of all the infrastructure (buildings, services, medical equipment, etc.) in the hospital must be folded into this. The cost per bed is an important consideration that will influence planned increases in capacity. At current costs, the capital cost of a bed varies between Rs. 5 lakh per bed for a basic community hospital in a rural setting, going up to Rs. 1 Cr per bed in a super-specialty hospital in a metro location. Considering we require beds at both ends of the spectrum, the key is to understand the mix of beds required. On that basis, the total expected cost can be arrived at. For a moment, let us assume that India has 1.4 beds per 1000 currently and this number should go up. Every addition of 0.1 beds per 1000 would mean a total addition of 140,000 beds. At the low end (Rs. 5 Lakhs per bed), this could require an outlay of Rs. 7,000 Crs, at the upper end, Rs. 140,000 Crs. In the absence of a data-driven approach to arrive at the mix, any estimate could be off the mark, and any plan based on such estimates could end up creating capacity that does not match requirements. In the past several decades, both the government and private sector have created additional hospital bed capacity independent of each other, and while there is still a significant demand-supply gap in our rural and semi-urban areas, we have ended up creating excess capacity in the urban and metro areas; in some instances even going past levels in countries with high per capita spending on healthcare. For instance, Bangalore city has 3.6 beds per 1000 population, ahead of New York City which has only three beds per 1000 population. Moreover, the occupancy rate across New York City hospital beds is around 75%, whereas most hospitals in Bangalore city are operating at under 60% occupancy rates, indicating an oversupply of hospital beds in Bangalore. In a situation where there is an excess supply of beds in the for-profit sector, the hospital owners respond by whipping up consumption, either through unnecessary hospitalization for minor conditions or extended stays.

Thereby, a potential loss to hospital owners is transmitted to patients who end up paying for superfluous consumption.

Who pays influences demand

The requirement for hospital beds is also influenced by who pays for their use. It is reasonable to expect that the demand for hospitalization from self-paying patients will be lower (the exception being high net-worth individuals who are preyed upon by for-profit hospitals to increase bed utilization) than from patients availing themselves of third-party payments like health insurance or employer-funded payments. Insurance penetration in India is low, despite the Ayushman Bharat program providing insurance coverage to many persons with low-income levels. The incidence of inpatient treatment (expressed as a percentage of the population seeking inpatient care) among the Ayushman Bharat beneficiaries at 1% is significantly lower than the incidence among persons with employer-provided or self-purchased health insurance plans, which is around 5.5%. This gap may be attributable to a lack of awareness of the Ayushman Bharat scheme as well as the fact that it covers only a subset of procedures. In the US, where insurance penetration is almost 97%, the incidence of hospitalization is ~ 10-12%. If we were to assume an overall 5.6% incidence rate in India (the incidence rate for individuals covered under employer-provided insurance) the arithmetic would be as follows:

S.No	Description	Nos	Units	Remarks/ explanations
Total Beds required for India under UHC				
	Current scenario			
1	India population	1408	Mil	in 2021
2	Current hospitalization incidence rate for insured persons	5.60%	%	
3	Therefore, total admissions/year if entire population had insurance	78.8	Mil	(1408*5.6%)
4	Average length of stay per admission	4	Days	
5	Therefore, Bed Days needed	315.4	Mil Bed Days	(78.8 M* 4 Days)
6	Hospital Service Days/year	300	Days	
7	Beds required at 100% Occupancy	1.05	Mil Beds	(315.4 Mil Bed Days/300 Days)
8	Beds required at 80% Occupancy	1.31	Mil Beds	
9	Beds per 1000 population	0.93	Beds/1000	(1.31*1000/1408)
	UHC Scenario			
1	Hospitalization incidence rate	8.40%	%	Bed use may go up by 50% under UHC
2	Total admissions/ year	118.27	Mil	(1408*8.4%)
3	Hospital Days	473.1	Mil Bed Days	(118.27 M*4 Days)
4	Beds required at 80% Occupancy	1.97	Mil	(473 Mil Bed Days/300 Days)
4a	Beds currently available	1.92	Mil	
5	Expressed as Beds required per 1000 population	1.4	Beds/1000	(1.97*1000/1408)

We have 1.4 beds per 1000, which matches the demand, as seen in the table, also at 1.4 beds per 1000. It is not so much a lack of beds, but the skewed distribution—with many metro areas having surplus bed capacity and rural areas having deficits. Most of the surplus in metro areas is overbuilt private hospital capacity. This could be usefully re-purposed to create focused care facilities where elective procedures can be done at scale. If we did this, the remaining gap in rural areas will be due to a deficit of emergency care beds and general hospital-type bed capacity. Substantial addition of emergency care outside metro areas will need to be created as a greenfield investment since such capacity does not presently exist. Expansion of bed capacity in district hospitals and the addition of bed capacity in the Comprehensive Care Centers can provide the 'solution shop' style capacity needed outside the major metros.

Intensive panic: Expanding Intensive Care Capacity

The second wave of COVID (April to May 2021) brought into stark relief the yawning gap that exists in the ability of our public healthcare institutions to provide critical and intensive care to large swathes of the Indian population. Even in the relatively well-provisioned major metros, many COVID patients died horrible deaths waiting for care outside large hospitals.

In April 2020, soon after the first wave was upon us, a group of researchers at the CDDEP (Center for Disease Dynamics, Economics and Policy), in collaboration with Princeton University, estimated the availability of total hospital beds and intensive care beds across the country. We provide in the table below data from a few of the larger states, along with a country-level comparison of the same ten countries we have selected for our tables.

S.No	State/Country	Popn Mil	Total Beds	Beds /1000	ICU beds	ICU Bed /1000
1	China	1433	7451600	5.20	52000	0.036
2	India	1366	1926060	1.41	95000	0.070
3	USA	328	908560	2.77	85000	0.258
4	Indonesia	260	306210	1.18	12975	0.050
5	Mexico	125	124900	1.0	4100	0.033
6	UK	67	163968	2.44	7100	0.105
7	Bangladesh	159	135405	0.85	1275	0.008
8	Nigeria	215	42960	0.20	650	0.003
9	Philippines	112	112100	1.00	4500	0.040
10	Canada	37	94170	2.58	4700	0.129
	Indian States					
1	Uttar Pradesh	221.5	206991	0.93	10350	0.05
2	Bihar	103.9	32623	0.31	1631	0.02
3	Andhra Pradesh	88.4	62803	0.71	3140	0.04
4	Tamil Nadu	69.7	210444	3.02	10522	0.15
5	Karnataka	68.4	189634	2.77	9482	0.14
6	Kerala	35.7	103154	2.89	5158	0.14
7	Jharkhand	33.2	29271	0.88	1464	0.04
8	Delhi	20.1	66182	3.29	3309	0.16

As seen in the table, the availability of ICU beds (expressed as beds per 1000 population) is around 0.07 for India, with wide state-to-state variability: as high as 0.15-0.16 in some of the southern states and as low as 0.02 in highly populated states like Bihar. ICU beds account for ~ 5% of total hospital beds.

Comparison with data from other countries provides some interesting insights. ICU bed availability in the US is 0.26 per 1000, which is ~ 4 times that in India. The availability of ICU beds in a 10 Km radius in the US is 2.7, which is a fourth of the India average of ~ 10. ICU beds in the US account for 9% of total hospital beds. The availability of ICU beds across OECD countries is 0.12 per 1000, which is comparable to figures for the Indian states in the south.

OECD countries have excellent transportation infrastructure and ambulance availability. Patients can be transported via road or air to reach a medical facility quickly. So even if ICU capacity were to be concentrated in a few locations, it would not be an issue. On the other hand, for a country like India where rural transportation infrastructure is still patchy, the availability of emergency and resuscitative care, near where people live, should be a priority.

The availability of ICU beds in India needs to be improved, alongside a more equitable geographical distribution of the same. If we were to benchmark against the OECD countries and use the average number rather than the highest, India should target 0.12 ICU beds per 1000. At the overall level, this could improve ICU bed availability per 10 km radius to over 15. In the process, the share of ICU beds in the total would go up to 7.8% from the current 5%. As we have argued elsewhere, there is no pressing need to increase overall hospital bed capacity in India. Additional ICU capacity can be created by upgrading regular hospital beds to provide critical care.

05 | DO WE NEED MORE DOCTORS?

"There is maladjustment in the distribution of trained personnel who congregate in urban areas owing to the lack of amenities and gainful employment in rural areas. Moreover, highly trained doctors of the medical profession are being utilized to carry out routine duties which can also be done by less qualified people. The need is to conserve such highly trained personnel for jobs that they ought to be doing, and to make greater use of auxiliary health personnel." - *Mudaliar Committee Report Recommendation (1962)*

Despite progress on several fronts, India continues to do poorly on measures of population health. One thing is abundantly clear—Indians need 'more' and 'better' healthcare. The call for 'more' healthcare is often translated as a need for more doctors. Doctors are a key ingredient in healthcare delivery. However, increasing the number of doctors will make a difference only if there is a shortage of doctors to start with.

Does India have a shortage of doctors?

Does India have a shortage of doctors? It depends on which part of the country you are in. Doctors are distributed unevenly, with some parts of the country having surpluses and some parts having extreme scarcity. This skew is prominent when comparing the availability of doctors in urban versus rural districts (the urban-to-rural doctor density ratio is 3.8:1). Seen in the aggregate, however, the number of doctors per 1000 population is 1.34, which exceeds the number prescribed by the WHO. So, the shortage is not one of numbers, it is one of distribution.

An absolute shortage of doctors, if it exists, is mainly in medical super-specialties like neurosurgery. Since most Indians cannot afford high-end super-specialist care and therefore do not seek such care, the shortage is not evident. It is a latent shortage that will become evident once the Government keeps its promise to provide free healthcare to all those who cannot afford it, whether under a system of Universal Health Coverage or something similar. Furthermore, high-end care is even more unevenly distributed, being concentrated mostly in rich metro regions. As a result, even the rural rich have to travel great distances to access the super specialty care they need.

The Government has made efforts to push medical care out into the rural hinterland in the form of Primary Health Centers. However, these outposts are under-equipped, understaffed, and unable to deliver anything more than the most rudimentary form of healthcare. In the meantime, the doctors who staff these medical outposts are limited to performing routine tasks, referring anything complex to colleagues in nearby towns. Over time, there is a downward spiral in their skill levels, leaving them unprepared to respond to medical emergencies needing immediate intervention. Even in the major metros, many general practitioners struggle to build their clientele, in the face of competition from super specialist colleagues, and suffer the same fate of skill obsolescence. Over time, many of them inevitably resort to generating income from kickbacks and referrals.

If we have fewer doctors in rural areas, will producing more doctors fix the problem? The assumption is that if we produce more doctors, some of them will spill over from the metro areas where there is a glut into smaller towns where there is a shortage. This assumption is a fallacy driven by the belief that healthcare, like any other economic activity, is bound by the same market forces: economic theory would state that as competition between doctors for the same patient pool grows, some of them will be driven to move to other areas that may be less attractive to their peers from a quality-of-living point of view. This ignores the reality of healthcare, in which information asymmetry between doctors and patients means that doctors have almost unlimited power to induce an increase in consumption. So, a doctor who sees fewer patients can compensate for a decline in income by prescribing an extra test, an extra medicine, or an extra procedure. This being the case, the production of additional doctors simply increases healthcare costs, with marginal utility or even a negative impact on the health of the population in areas already oversupplied with doctors. The quality-of-life difference between rural and urban environments is a gap that cannot be bridged simply by creating more doctors.

While it may be questionable if we have a deficit of doctors, it is a fact that healthcare delivery to large segments of the population is insufficient both in quantity and quality. So, if we do not train more doctors, what can we do to solve this issue? There are at least three things we ought to look at before we expand capacity in medical colleges and train more doctors. First, many of the things that front-line doctors do today as part of their medical duties can easily be performed by community health workers. This includes everything from doing basic physical exams to treating minor conditions. We can deploy trained community health workers in rural areas. They can be tethered via tele-health linkages to doctor colleagues who can back them up when necessary. It is workable to have such health workers even in remote regions, providing care that is lacking today. A cadre of trained community health workers deployed in Chhattisgarh and Assam has shown that this system works very well and can replace doctors for many of the tasks that doctors currently perform[12].

Second, we should broaden the skills of existing front-line doctors to include a wider range of procedures so that they can take on higher-value care. Again, front-line doctors can be supported by experts using tele-health bridges to the nearest large medical center. Continuing medical education and short-term certification courses can be a means to upgrade the skill levels of front-line doctors so that they deliver high-value care.

Third, we must devise mechanisms for existing pools of doctors concentrated in large cities to move to tier 2 and 3 towns. The socioeconomic factors underlying the attraction of large metros are hard to match. However, solo practitioners in big cities who are being muscled out by organized players may find it attractive to move to smaller towns if given the option to work in communal settings, such as group practices. Comprehensive Health Centers where they have access to a wider and deeper range of resources, including diagnostic equipment and specialist colleagues on whom they can rely for supplemental expertise and a collegial work environment, can be a magnet to attract solo practitioners from large cities to smaller towns.

We definitely need more healthcare workers.

These suggestions do not call for training more doctors, but they certainly call for training a cadre of healthcare workers—community health workers—who are deployed on the front lines of healthcare and who can take up a substantial part of the workload of front-line doctors. That will free up doctors and allow them to focus on the more complex pieces of healthcare commensurate with the cost incurred in training them. The challenge that remains, therefore, will be the problem of training community health workers in large numbers. This problem can be solved more easily and cost-effectively compared to training doctors. More importantly, this cadre can be sourced from the talent pool in villages, ensuring that they are acclimatized to serving near their homes. This could also have the spin-off benefit of creating large-scale skilled employment opportunities for the rural poor.

What can we do with the doctors who are currently performing low-value front-line tasks? They have to be up-skilled to perform minor procedures and surgery, which, although part of the training of an MBBS doctor, are skills that are quickly lost due to disuse. They can then cover for the looming shortages of doctors that will only worsen as more patients access such care through schemes like Ayushman Bharat.

The pandemic has brought to public attention the inadequacies in Indian public healthcare. The Government's placating response is to build more medical colleges and turn out more doctors. The plight of Indian medical students returning from Ukraine has played into the myth that we have too few doctors and inadequate capacity to train the numbers we need. While the stark numbers reported in our public health scorecard are objective reality, the inference that training more doctors will solve the issue is a fantasy. We do not simply need more doctors of the kind we have already. We need better trained doctors doing higher value work. In select super specialties, we may need to train more specialists to handle the consequences of emerging epidemics of lifestyle disease. But mostly what we need is a well-integrated system of healthcare where tele-health-enabled front-line healthcare workers can satisfy the demand for low-value healthcare closer to where the patients live, thus stopping the large-scale migration of the sick to the cities where they add to the burden of our already stretched public health infrastructure. We now describe the kind of "tech-enabled" healthcare worker who can fill the gap.

The tech-enabled healthcare worker

Primary healthcare is the backbone of any healthcare system: it provides comprehensive, longitudinal, and coordinated care that holds together the fragmented components of healthcare, including care delivered by specialists to whom the primary care physician may refer a patient. It also provides opportunities to screen for chronic lifestyle diseases like hypertension and diabetes that can smolder undetected for decades before causing symptoms. India's intended move to Universal Health Coverage (UHC) is predicated on access to high-quality primary healthcare. However, achieving universal primary healthcare coverage remains a distant dream. Rural areas where 70% of the Indian population lives have only 34% of India's doctors. It takes six years to train a doctor. Even if we could magically conjure up doctors, it is unlikely that it will make a significant difference to the rural needs anytime soon, since the newly minted doctors will also want to reside and practice in urban areas.

The problem of access to primary healthcare is not a new one. One commonly employed response in many countries has been to deploy

Community Health Workers (CHWs) who can provide the basic minimum health needs. India has already deployed one of the largest cadres of community healthcare workers in the world—the ASHA (Accredited Social Health Activist) worker (estimated to be around 1.0 million in position). However, ASHA workers are considered volunteers and have operated at the fringes of the formal healthcare system. Although they have had an impact on maternal and child care, they have not achieved the status of being viewed as the front-line for the formal primary healthcare system. The Indian primary healthcare system is absent in many villages, and even when it is present, it is hardly up to the task of providing comprehensive preventive and wellness care. As a result, most primary healthcare in villages is delivered by informal practitioners who have no formal qualifications or training, except maybe some experience working with a doctor or a pharmacist in a nearby town.

India's modest accomplishment with the ASHA cadre is not a reflection of the enormous possibilities inherent in the use of CHWs to deliver front-line primary care. Brazil has created a cadre of community health workers who are trained to a level where they can deliver most of the care that a doctor in primary care delivers (11). In addition, they are integrated with the primary healthcare team and serve as a bridge between communities and the health system. The CHWs in Brazil (~ 1.2 per 1000 population) make monthly household visits during which they follow up and assist longitudinally with routine preventive screening and chronic health conditions. One advantage of CHWs in Brazil is the fact that they are recruited from within the community and deliver care by visiting the homes in their locality.

It will be a good first step to upgrade India's ASHA workers to a level similar to the CHWs in Brazil. Beyond this, there is a unique opportunity to create a disruptive model of technology-enabled healthcare that India is superbly equipped to execute. And the time may be ripe to create a world-leading model of technology-enabled front-line healthcare. Some of the key ingredients to support such an initiative are already being put in place in the form of digital tools like UHID (Unique Health Identification) and the other components of the National Health Stack. Bandwidth on mobile networks is improving with the ongoing implementation of 5G networks, even in peri-urban areas. India has already proven its capabilities in rolling out large-scale digitally enabled programs, as we saw during the COVID-19 pandemic when India implemented a model for vaccination scheduling and certification. India also has a vibrant startup health technology sector that is not only producing tools for digital engagement but also affordable point-of-care devices. This can be the substratum for a bold initiative to produce 1 million plus tech-enabled front-line healthcare workers over the next 5-10 years, who can deliver primary healthcare to the homes of the rural population living in the farthest reaches. Let us, for now, call them Tech-enabled Healthcare Workers (THWs).

THWs should be certified health workers trained to perform many common front-line procedures (like intravenous injections and suture removal) and diagnostic tests. They will be electronically tethered to the nearest primary health center via a smartphone. They will be equipped with smartphone apps that will help them capture patient details on an electronic medical record, triage patients, initiate tele-health sessions with doctors when needed, and schedule in-person visits to the doctor at the nearest primary health center. The Electronic Health Records (EHRs) will be available to patients on basic smartphones and shareable using secure gateway mechanisms. By using a variety of Point of Care tools including everything from basic BP measurements to glucose and hemoglobin measurements, as well as portable devices that can capture retinal images and even fetal monitors, the THWs will be in a position to deliver almost all the care that is available at a PHC.

Beyond routine health needs, THWs can also be trained to provide resuscitative care (care given to stabilize a patient who can subsequently be moved to an acute care facility). Prompt provision of resuscitative care can be the game changer in improving clinical outcomes for vast numbers of suddenly acutely ill patients who live in regions where acute care is not available in the vicinity. THWs can provide immediate and urgent care, e.g., a thrombolytic for stroke or a snake antivenom, or an antiepileptic for uncontrolled seizures or stopping uncontrolled bleeding from a wound, etc., with guidance provided through a tele-health device.

India also faces an acute and growing shortage of trained nurses. Against an OECD average of around eight nurses per 1000 population, India has only 1.8 nurses per 1000. Trained nurses are also fleeing for foreign shores, attracted by the compensation and greater respect the nursing profession receives in those countries. If we are to reach OECD levels of nurse numbers, we will have to train an additional 9 million nurses, which may take 30 years given that we only train about 3.5 lakh nurses per year. THWs trained like nurses on performing procedures but without the deep training in basic and clinical sciences could be a useful resource to not only fill the gap in the supply of nurses but also mitigate physician shortages by relieving doctors of routine tasks that can easily be undertaken by a THW.

THWs will cost a lot more than ASHA workers. But they will also deliver a lot more value in terms of timely, high-quality healthcare at the doorstep of citizens. We estimate the cost of deploying a million THWs to be an annual charge of around INR 60,000 crore. But if such a system could reduce disability from chronic diseases by 30% and hospitalization instances by another 30%, then the cost can easily be recovered.

Primary Healthcare is unable to deliver on its promise even in developed countries like the UK, where a shortage of doctors and the administrative complexity of the referral system to get specialist attention leads to long delays in care. We, in India, are starting with a clean slate. Most of our investments in UHC are in the future. We have to be prudent in allocating these investments in a manner that can realistically produce high-quality healthcare at an affordable cost. India's unique combination of problems of huge scale co-located with the capability to develop scalable technology-enabled solutions is an opportunity we cannot miss. Through the deployment of a large-scale

THW program, the Government can deliver healthcare that can be the envy even of many first-world nations while generating the centripetal forces that drive tech innovation from India into the heart of healthcare. And since our problems may be large but not unique, the solutions that India innovates can be replicated and deployed across the world, giving India the status of a leader in solving some of the most intractable healthcare problems faced by all nations today.

Finally, we need at least one million technology-enabled healthcare workers. The need for such workers will grow with the aging of the population. This is a need not just in India. Across the world, the same demographic trends are playing out, with India only now catching up. If we can train several million THWs, then some of them are also likely to find well-paying jobs in health systems in other countries. This could be the solution to the youth unemployment problem that is only likely to get worse when home delivery workers get displaced by drones, drivers by autonomous vehicles, and IT professionals by the tools of AI/ML. The job of the THW may be one of the fastest-expanding job categories in the future for which India can be a major supplier of trained talent.

06 | COMPLETING THE ECOSYSTEM

We have talked about primary health care and hospitals. A healthcare ecosystem is composed of a multitude of other players, and we will now turn our attention briefly to some of them.

One of the critical areas of need in any healthcare ecosystem is emergency and acute care. There is a small window period from the onset of a heart attack, a stroke, or a snake bite when tissue damage is largely reversible. This has been referred to as the golden period. Getting a patient to the hospital within the golden period has a positive impact on outcomes. Most Indians do not live close enough to a hospital to get timely emergency care. For a country where a majority of the population lives in villages, it may be a while before every corner has reasonable access to emergency care. Without such access, Universal Health Coverage would be incomplete. So, how do we assure citizens that they will have access to emergency care during the golden period?

One way to achieve this is to detach Emergency Care from large hospitals and make standalone emergency care mini-hospitals more widely available. Such emergency medical centers can be established within a 5-10 KM distance from any place in India. They should be equipped with ambulances that can cover a 10 KM radius in 20-30 minutes. This can be achieved by locating them close to major highways. A 20-30 minute one-way journey means that an ambulance can reach an emergency patient well within one hour, and if the ambulance is suitably equipped, some forms of emergency care can be initiated at the same time that the patient is picked up. For a country the size of India, some 1000 such emergency medical centers may be needed. This is a large but manageable task that can be achieved over some time.

In the meantime, with the use of tele-health in the hands of village-level community health workers, it should be possible to deliver basic emergency care even in remote regions that are more than 10 KM away from the nearest emergency center. Such care can consist of CPR, intravenous medications including thrombolytics, anti-asthmatics and anti-epileptics, defibrillation, intravenous fluids, airway maintenance, and other such means to stabilize the patient and extend the golden period until the patient can be moved to a nearby emergency medical center. A nationwide network of emergency care centers and community health workers trained to handle basic emergencies with support from tele-health could have made a significant difference during the recent pandemic. The critical piece here is training the CHW in emergency care and ensuring that they have 24/7 access via tele-health technology to expert emergency care-trained physicians who can guide them on treatment.

Even with the coverage being as broad as it is in this book, we have left out very important aspects that should be covered in the design of a healthcare ecosystem. For example, there is much more we could say about public health and preventive health concepts. This includes things like designing workplaces and living spaces to accommodate the need for physical activity. And then there is the need for providing healthy nutritional choices—easier said than done in an environment saddled with inexpensive and super convenient processed food choices. A lot could be said about using behavioral nudges to drive healthy lifestyle choices, e.g., having walk-only central business districts in cities. We really cannot make a big dent in our healthcare problems without addressing these elephants in the room. In this book, we have chosen to reduce the span of coverage to focus on issues where the answers are not so simple or readily available. We do this intentionally so that we are addressing complex problems with innovative and simple solutions that are feasible and realistic in the near term and yet are not the subject of conversation simply because they are seen as complex and 'wicked' problems with no easy solutions in sight.

Our design and the existing ecosystem

How does what we propose compare to the ecosystem as it exists today? On the face of it, our proposal is radical. However, there are recognizable elements of the current ecosystem in what we have proposed.

India's public healthcare system as it is now can be categorized into primary, secondary, and tertiary levels. The primary level comprises sub-centers and PHCs, which are the first points of contact between the community and the public healthcare system and form the foundation of India's public healthcare.

In the current system, a sub-center serves a population of 3,000 in hilly/hard-to-reach/tribal areas and a population of 5,000 in plains. Sub-centers are staffed with at least one auxiliary nurse midwife/female health worker and one male health worker.

In the ecosystem we envision, an up-skilled Community Health Worker equipped with point-of-care and tele-health technologies will be the primary and first point of contact for the community. The CHW will staff the upgraded equivalent of the sub-center.

In the current ecosystem, the Primary Health Center (PHC) is a referral unit for six sub-centers and is the first point of contact between the village community and a medical officer. It serves a population of 20,000 in hilly/hard-to-reach/tribal areas and 30,000 in plain areas. It should be staffed by a minimum of a medical officer supported by 14 paramedical and other staff such as nurses, a laboratory technician, and a pharmacist. Furthermore, it has 4–6 beds. Its goal is to provide integrated, curative, and preventive healthcare to the rural population, with an emphasis on preventive and promotive care.

Community Health Center (CHC): The secondary level of healthcare comprises CHCs and smaller sub-district hospitals. A CHC acts as a referral unit for PHCs and serves a population of 80,000 in hilly/hard-to-reach/ tribal areas and 120,000 in plain areas. A CHC must have four medical specialists: a surgeon, a physician, a gynecologist and a pediatrician with 21 paramedical and other staff. It is supposed to have 30 beds, an operating theater, an X-ray, a labor room, and laboratory facilities.

In the system we envision the Primary Health Center, and the Community Health center are rolled into one, what we call the Comprehensive Community-Care Center (CCC) which is staffed by a "Comprehensive Care Physician" or "Comprehensivist" along with specialists available for interventional treatment for common NCDs, either permanently located in the CCC or rotating through nearby hospitals.

The tertiary level of healthcare includes district/general hospitals, medical colleges, and super-specialty hospitals under both government and private providers.

These will be replaced in the ecosystem we have laid out by Emergency Acute Care Hospitals, Focused Care Hospitals, Para-Hospitals, and Multi-speciality General - teaching and training Hospitals.

In the section on UHC, we discuss the business models that enmesh public and private players to create the system that we envision.

Healthcare journeys in the ecosystem

In order to envision what the ecosystem we propose will deliver, we describe several hypothetical scenarios.

Scenario 1: Ashok is a farmworker. He works in a remote village several hours away from the nearest Comprehensive Care Center. Ashok suffers a snakebite in the field. He uses his phone to call Bhushan, the village Community Health Worker. The CHW shows up and transports Ashok to the village health center using a bike ambulance. At the village health center, there is a refrigerator containing snake antivenom effective against the common venomous snakes of the region. After a quick consultation over the tele-health system with the doctor at the nearby Emergency Care Center, Bhushan administers the antivenom and keeps

Ashok under observation. Due to the timely administration of the antivenom, Ashok does not need hospitalization and can return home.

Scenario 2: Rukmini, a villager, is pregnant. Rani, the local community health worker, has her electronic medical records on her smartphone UHC app and follows up on her clinical status diligently, especially because she has pregnancy-induced hypertension. A month before her due date, Rukmini experiences some abdominal pain and calls Rani to check on her. Rani visits Rukmini, and after conducting a general physical examination, she connects via her tele-health device with the Comprehensive Care Center. The obstetrician there advises an ultrasound and tocography. Rani has portable versions of both devices and quickly transmits the data to the obstetrician via the tele-health system. The obstetrician reviews the data alongside Rukmini's past records using the EHR platform and determines that there is no need to worry. Rukmini is reassured and advised to stay put. She has a normal delivery a month later.

Scenario 3: Ashok is a shopkeeper near a small town. He has diabetes and hypertension for which he is receiving treatment. One day, he notices that his legs are swollen. He goes to the nearest Comprehensive Care Center to see his regular health worker, John, whom he has been seeing for the past ten years. John quickly checks Ashok's record, asks Ashok a few questions about his complaint, conducts a detailed physical examination, and orders a couple of blood tests as per the recommendation of the electronic treatment algorithm on his phone. The blood test results are available in 30 minutes, and John accompanies Ashok to see his assigned physician, Dr. Kumar. Dr. Kumar reviews the data collected by John, reviews the EHR where the blood test results are already available, checks a few clinical parameters, and decides that Ashok needs to be seen by a nephrologist. Using his electronic calendar, he schedules a visit for Ashok to the nephrologist after three days. The nephrologist reviews Ashok's situation along with John and decides that his kidney function status does not require immediate dialysis and advises some dietary changes and tighter glucose control. He notes this in the EHR and sends Ashok back to Dr. Kumar for further management and follow-up.

Scenario 4: Mahima is 63 years old and has had chronic joint pain in her left knee for the past 8 years. She is being treated with medicines at the nearby Comprehensive Care Center, although she has to visit them only once or twice a year since Majid, the CHW, is able to help her with her medications, and once in a while brings in a doctor on his tele-health device to advise on issues that he is not trained to handle. But this time, Mahima's pain is beyond control with medications, and from her record, Majid knows that she has osteoarthritis and is due for a knee replacement. Majid asks her to go to the Comprehensive Care Center, where her physician sees her and schedules her for a knee replacement facility at the nearest Joint Replacement Focused Care Facility. On the scheduled date, Mahima shows up at the Focused Care Facility along with all the test results prescribed for approval for surgery. She is admitted, and the surgery is done the same day. The same evening, she is shifted to a nearby Step-Down hospital where family members accompanying the patient are trained on post-op rehabilitation, and nurses provide monitoring. Resident doctors provide medical support, as required, and if complications arise, they can call specialists on call at the Focused Care Facility. Fortunately, Mahima's recovery is uneventful, which is not surprising, considering that the Joint Replacement Focused Care Facility where she underwent the surgery performs the largest number of such operations anywhere in the world, and their staff is trained to such perfection they can almost do everything with their eyes closed. They also publish the results of their work and the innovations they have introduced in prestigious medical journals like The Lancet. In addition they regularly host meetings for visiting surgeons to learn the techniques and processes they have innovated to do Joint Replacement at 1/30th the cost of any other center in the world with results that are superior by 30-50%. Mahima walks home after a month, fully recovered and cheerful, knowing that she can be active and lose some of the weight she had put on.

This last part may sound fanciful, but it is not. Extraordinary results of a similar nature have been achieved by Aravind Eye Care that are now widely publicized. Before Aravind, a hand surgeon at a Government Hospital in Chennai ran one of the worlds largest hand reconstructive surgery centers with results that impressed visiting surgeons from OECD countries[13].

SECTION SUMMARY AND CONCLUSIONS

Let us start by recapping some facts:

1. The best-known examples of high-quality healthcare anywhere in the world are focused care facilities, like Shouldice Hernia Hospital in Canada and Aravind Eye Care in India.

2. The average time primary care physicians in India spend in consultations is around 2 minutes. In Canada, it is around 15 minutes, and in Sweden, around 22 minutes.

3. Community Health Workers deliver similar or better care compared to traditional physician-delivered healthcare in rural regions of India.

4. India has 1.8 nurses per 1000 population. In countries with high UHC scores like Australia, Canada, and the UK, there are at least seven nurses per 1000 population. Richer countries typically have 2.5 to 3 times as many nurses as doctors. At current levels of nurse education, between now and 2030, India could potentially reach a level of 3.5 nurses per 1000. To reach a level of 7, India would need to train triple the number of nurses trained per year (~1.0 million per year, against the current capacity of 3.5 lakh per year).

Healthcare is like an orchestra. When healthcare is great, it will be no less than a symphony played by the orchestra. The orchestra needs a conductor who understands each instrument, knows the strengths of each member of the orchestra, and knows how to get the best out of them in the service of music. The role of the conductor for healthcare is played by the Comprehensive Care Team (the nomenclature we use for our upgraded version of Primary Healthcare) - the first point where the patient reaches out for relief. This team, which includes the Comprehensive Care Physician or Comprehensivist, then swings into action to conscript and coordinate the various components of healthcare that can provide high-quality relief for the patient. Both accountability and responsibility are shifted to this core. This upturns the current hierarchical model where specialists sit at the top. In the model we propose, the Comprehensive Care Team is at the core, orchestrating the activities of the specialties while being the first and primary responders to patient needs. The exceptions will be emergencies and the episodes when the patient is under the direct care of a specialist. Even in hospitals, a cadre of what has been called "hospitalists" in the US can serve a coordinating function that complements the role of the Comprehensive Care Physician.

Emergency healthcare will focus on providing urgent care and stabilizing the patient until the acute episode has passed. Subsequent long-term care, such as rehabilitation after acute trauma or a heart attack, may involve transferring the patient to a chronic care facility (of the focused care or general care kind) before stepping them down and eventually discharging them to home care. This is where the Comprehensive Care concept kicks in. It will not only provide a whole suite of care components but also recruit community members as Community Health Workers to provide local context-relevant continuous care.

By segregating care between focused care institutions and solution shop-style institutions, we will improve the quality of care at both ends. Focused care facilities will render high-quality, protocol driven care at scale, thus bringing down costs, while the solution shop institutions will provide complex multispecialty attention that is often required for patients with multi-organ disease, rare conditions, or difficult-to-diagnose conditions. The latter should ideally be teamed up with teaching hospitals and medical colleges, as well as research laboratories pioneering next-generation treatments.

We have proposed a system whereby key components that are operated (not necessarily owned) by the Government act as the tree trunk from which the legacy hodgepodge of models and assets can branch, without losing the benefits that result from a well-integrated system. The "ideal" ecosystem we have crafted is vastly different enough from what exists today. We need to find a route from the current state to this end state that is not disruptive in the short term. This is a matter for discussion and debate.

HEALTHCARE DOWN THE DRAIN

The proportion of healthcare expenditure that is wasted is estimated to be as high as 50%. This is a scandal that is well known to insiders, but poorly appreciated by those outside the system. Unless we fix this, any increase in spending on healthcare will simply get sucked out of the system as waste.

Though the doctors treated him, let his blood, and gave him medications to drink, he nevertheless recovered.

    - Leo Tolstoy, War and Peace

…if nothing is done to make the system more efficient—better cost control, better coverage, better access, better quality of care—health care, like Pac-Man, will simply continue to chew up more and more of the American economy.

    —Uwe Reinhardt

"Americans spend almost 40% more per capita for health care than any other country, yet rank 27th in infant mortality, 27th in life expectancy, and are less satisfied with their care than the English, Canadians, or Germans. Serious medication errors occur in 7 of 100 hospital admissions, and more than 80000 unnecessary hysterectomies and 500000 unnecessary cesarean deliveries are performed in this country each year. Only 1 in 5 elderly myocardial infarction survivors receive appropriate medications to reduce the risks of recurrence, and even fewer high-risk elderly individuals are vaccinated against pneumococcus. Extensive waits and delays abound in health care, far more than individuals tolerate in other service sectors."

Donald Berwick, in "Disseminating Innovations in Health Care"

01 | HEALTHCARE AND WASTE

Healthcare is already expensive and growing increasingly so. Large numbers of Indians struggle for access to healthcare due to a lack of public health facilities and the absence of insurance coverage. Despite the fact that healthcare is already unaffordable for many, the sad fact is that as much as 50% of the money we spend on healthcare is wasted. This money is wasted either because it does not help or, even worse, it jeopardizes health, thereby increasing healthcare costs.

Why is so much spending on healthcare wasted?

The prevailing fee-for-service model in private healthcare encourages consumption; the time a doctor spends on seeing a patient is a cost to her. But there is no cost to her if she simply orders some tests. Instead of taking a detailed history and conducting a physical examination that could help arrive at a diagnosis, she is incentivized to send you away for tests. She may also derive a commission from the price you pay for the tests. In her mind, she may justify unnecessary testing by saying that it is needed to arrive at a definitive diagnosis, and therefore, why waste time on history taking and physical exams? This is the slippery road that leads to higher healthcare costs. Notably, tests can be fallible and lead to costly cycles of more testing and wrong treatment.

There is an additional twist in this tale. A significant proportion of hospital treatment in private hospitals is paid for by third-party insurers. In such cases, there is no incentive for the patient to even care about the cost of care. It is simply a negotiation between the insurer and the hospital, which the hospital often wins because of the asymmetric availability of information.

There are plenty of gray zones in medicine—situations that are not clearly black or white. In such situations, the doctor has to make a judicious call based on experience. Treatment decisions in these gray zones are influenced by external factors, resulting in treatment choices that are useless or even downright harmful to the patient. For example, doctors may be conditioned by their need to look good against the competition, and so quickly adopting newfangled and unproven technologies. Such tendencies are amplified by the additional income doctors can earn from such choices.

Compounding these issues is the opacity that obscures the work of doctors. Even if the patient is fully informed, the average patient cannot act as a self-interested agent since the information about her health and the numerous possible treatment options is too complex to digest. Finally, the fragmentation of medical care resulting from the proliferation of super-specialties atomizes and disperses the decision process on treatment choices in such a manner that even a physician will find it a challenge to pull all the information together into a comprehensible whole. In the resulting ungovernable chaotic mess, it is impossible to untangle justifiable from unjustifiable consumption and costs.

Examples of waste

Although it may be readily apparent to anyone who has experienced healthcare in India what we mean by waste, fraud, and error, a few illustrative examples may be helpful, especially since the three are so intertwined.

You go to a pediatrician for your child who has a fever and a sore throat. He checks her and sees all the signs of an acute viral infection. Nevertheless, he prescribes antibiotics. He does this systematically in the community he serves. Soon, resistant bacterial strains emerge as a result of antibiotic overuse, and elders in the community start dying of infections from resistant organisms. Waste?

Your uncle goes to a cardiologist for chest congestion. Your uncle also suffers from heart failure and an abnormal heart rhythm that is controlled with drugs. The cardiologist determines that the cause is allergic and prescribes an antihistamine that should not be given along with the other drug. There is a drug interaction between the antihistamine and the drug given for the abnormal rhythm. Your uncle has a cardiac arrest. The cause is diagnosed too late, and he dies in the hospital several days later. Error?

A cousin is admitted to the hospital for a heart condition. It is easily controlled with medication. But while you are waiting outside the ICU, a junior doctor sizes you up and suggests a costly internal pacemaker procedure, for which the doctor receives a cut from the pacemaker manufacturer. Fraud?

Yet another emotionally fraught example experienced by patients at the bottom of the income pyramid: a nurse compels a mother to pay a fee to see her newborn girl — a higher charge had the baby been a boy. Corruption?

Is dishing out expensive and unneeded treatments for those who can afford them a victimless crime? For example, a dying patient in the ICU in the last few hours of life is prescribed a panel of expensive tests and treatments that are futile. This is both fraud and waste. But if the family can afford the extra cost, is it victimless? No, it is not. Apart from the costs to the family of the patient from such unnecessary treatment, there is also the societal cost of consumption of resources that might have been productively applied to the life of a person who needed the treatment but could not afford it.

Each of the examples above is inextricably linked with the other two strands in this reinforcing cord that we call WaFEr - Waste, Fraud, and Error. For example, putting a pacemaker in someone who does not need it is an example of waste. While in the example given above, the pacemaker was not needed, there are many gray areas where the correct decision is not so obvious. In such cases, the cat on the wall can be made to jump to either side, depending on available incentives. A financial incentive can encourage a cardiologist to put in place a stent, although the use of the stent may fall in the category of a gray zone intervention where it is not clear if it is needed. What do you think the doctor will do in such a situation? He will simply act in his own interest by putting in a stent if he receives a commission on the price of the stent. And he will also, most likely, put in the most expensive stent that is on offer.

Health Innovation and Waste

Many new-age business models are less about delivering value generating healthcare and more about parasitically capturing inefficiencies in patient spending from existing players. While this does lead to a leaner marketplace, it also makes for a meaner marketplace where patient interests and clinical outcomes are sidelined in the pursuit of opportunistic revenue diversion. An example: milking excess capacity in healthcare systems in the form of underutilized operating rooms by asking patients to undergo procedures that are not needed, such as hysterectomy (uterus removal), even when there is no medical indication.

Technological advancements in medicine will continue to produce innovations that offer great benefits to some patients but can easily be overused in others. Healthcare systems must be designed to foster innovation and promote its use in patients for whom the benefits can be justified. We may need a specialized agency, like the National Institute for Clinical Excellence in the UK, to perform risk-benefit calculations based on which treatments can be targeted to those who will benefit from them, rather than being wasted on those for whom the benefit does not justify the cost. This will become even more important with the arrival of expensive new treatments like cell and gene therapy.

There is, as yet, little evidence of comparative effectiveness for a vast array of treatments. For example, for most cancers, proton-beam therapy may not offer any advantage over conventional approaches. Innovations are not always improvements over older treatment approaches. For example, bioabsorbable cardiac stents were found to be inferior or at best equal to older and cheaper stent technologies. Moreover, many drug studies compare new drugs to placebos, rather than conducting "head-to-head" comparisons with other drugs on the market, thus, failing to generate evidence on whether the new drug is any better than older treatments.

02 | DE-WAFERING HEALTHCARE

Waste, **F**raud, and **Er**ror (WaFEr) are leeches that bleed healthcare. Unless we fix them, spending more money on healthcare will be like dousing a flame with petrol.

Our low GDP per capita caps our ability to spend on healthcare

Discussions about the need to move toward Universal Health Coverage (UHC) center around the subject of how much money we should spend as a percentage of GDP. Comparisons are drawn with other countries that deliver UHC. The comparison is problematic since India, with its large population, has a proportionally larger GDP. Although GDP per capita, a better measure of the ability to spend on services for individual citizens, is comparatively low (USD 2099 for India versus USD 43000 for the UK). A more apt calculation is—what percent of GDP per capita can we spend on healthcare? When we do the math, we find that we need to raise spending to 71% of GDP per capita to match in absolute terms what the UK (whose National Health Service is an oft cited paragon among UHC models) spends per capita on healthcare (even after adjusting for purchasing power). Clearly we cannot afford UHC the way we deliver healthcare now.

We need to increase productivity in healthcare

We need to look at alternative ways to fund the incremental spending, and one obvious way is to make healthcare spending more productive. The investment required to generate a desired Clinical Outcome is one way of measuring productivity in healthcare. For example, if we take the Infant Mortality Rate (IMR) as a sample metric, how much additional spending do we need to put in to achieve a 10% reduction in IMR? The costs that go into healthcare are obvious—wages of healthcare workers, cost of capital on building and equipment, and so on. Buried in this is a hidden cost that remains unmeasured and unconsidered. What is this hidden cost? This is the cost resulting from unchecked Waste, Fraud, and Errors in healthcare delivery.

Waste, Fraud, and Error are inextricably intertwined

Fraud increases waste, and waste can spur fraud. Similarly, fraud can result in errors, and errors can result in waste. We can illustrate this by expanding on the example cited above. Doctor X, responding to incentives (bribes) from pharmaceutical industry representatives, "over prescribes" an expensive new class of antibiotics. Over time, bugs develop resistance, requiring even more expensive antibiotics and treatment in intensive care. While prescribing unneeded antibiotics to earn a kickback from the pharma company is an example of fraud, the adverse consequence for patients can be considered iatrogenic or physician-induced and therefore an example of error. The Herculean efforts and costs to manage the unleashed epidemic of antibiotic resistance are examples of waste that could have been avoided. In other words, there are no watertight compartments sealing off the three sins of waste, fraud, and error.

Cost of WaFEr in India

There are no systematic studies of WaFEr in Indian healthcare, but we estimate, based on data from other countries and patches of data available for India, that the cost of WaFEr is around INR 80,000 Crs. It may not be possible to eliminate this. However, with the right checks in place, we can bring this down by as much as 50%. The resulting INR 40,000 Crs in savings can subsidize high-quality healthcare for all citizens as part of Universal Health Coverage.

An example of WaFEr that is easily fixed

The lowest hanging fruit in the context of WaFEr is the use of branded medicines when equivalent generic medicines can do the job. Shifting to generic medicines at scale is not a new idea—it was proposed by the Indian Government in 2014. Branded medicines and their generic equivalents are exact replicas. A memorable brand name merely adds cosmetic value and is intended as a mnemonic for doctors; a constant nudge to prescribe the brand. For that cosmetic difference, the patient pays a huge premium. For example, the popular cholesterol-lowering drug known by its generic name as Atorvastatin is known as Atorva when sold by Zydus Pharma and as Lipikind when sold by Mankind Pharma and simply as Atorvastatin when sold by the low-price Jan Aushadhi Pharmacies[1]. The respective prices for a 10 mg tablet are INR 9.18, INR 3.69, and INR 0.56. There is a 16-fold difference between the top brand and the generic. Would you accept a 16-fold difference in the price of a commodity like wheat flour or salt? Then why do customers accept this difference? Simply because the role of prescriber and payer is separated. The doctor chooses the brand that rewards him, and the patient has to go along since she cannot act otherwise without offending the doctor (the dispensing pharmacist and the doctor often work in nexus since the pharmacist also gains from dispensing the higher-margin drug).

The only way to break through this is to ban the branding of medicines altogether and identify medicines only by their generic name. Companies can be allowed to tag their company names after the name of the generic ingredient, e.g., Atorvastatin-Zydus or Atorvastatin-Mankind, just so that there is sufficient skin in the game for pharma companies to ensure product quality. In one stroke, multiple intertwined sins can be eliminated: "over-prescribing," doctor kickbacks, and "mis-prescribing" due to confusingly similar brand names. A big bite can also be taken from the healthcare bill—about INR 10,000 to 15,000 crore is an estimate.

Going generic will boost innovation and quality

Going generic cold turkey will be easy to legislate, but there will be pain, as many subscale pharma companies will shut down, and marketing jobs will be lost. The long-term benefits will, however, outweigh the short-term pain. Pharma companies will be forced to innovate since a brand name will no longer offer a moat for their products. Jobs in research and development and regulatory science will grow. There will also be an improvement in drug quality (ever wondered why the US FDA pulls up Indian companies so very often, whereas the Indian drug regulator seems to see nothing fishy at all?) since that will be the only differentiator distinguishing different versions of a generic drug.

Eliminating WaFEr has to underpin ambitious plans to implement UHC

Eliminating WaFEr from the practice of medicine has to be a journey with many incremental steps. But the reward is not just financial. Eliminating WaFEr improves the quality of healthcare.

A critical tool enabling the elimination of WaFEr is transparency on prices and clinical outcomes, combined with a gatekeeper function for primary healthcare and a shift from fee-based to value-based healthcare. Elimination of WaFEr calls for informed and attentive regulatory oversight by the Government. Remunerating public healthcare workers adequately, ensuring social accountability, and building transparency are key. This calls for increased Government spending on public health, not simply in building more hospitals, but wrapping the infrastructure in an envelope of good Governance. The cost saved from eliminating WaFer will more than compensate for this increased expenditure on good Governance. Going completely generic on medicines and devices may be a good place to start the de-WaFEring process.

De-WaFEring healthcare can be a tremendous opportunity to bring down healthcare costs. A mix of tightly enforced regulations can be used to do this. In an environment where resources have to be stretched to meet the objective of UHC, eliminating WaFEr is a necessary first step.

TABLE: List of procedures found to be wasteful (as per the US Lown Institute Hospitals Index[2]):

1. **Arthroscopic knee surgery** – Surgery to remove damaged cartilage or bone in the knee using an arthroscope (tiny camera). Defined as overuse for patients with osteoarthritis or "runner's knee" (damaged cartilage). Excluding patients with meniscal tears.

2. **Carotid artery imaging for fainting** – A test to screen for carotid (neck) artery disease. Considered overuse for patients where syncope (fainting) is the primary diagnosis, and there is no history of syncope in the past two years. Excluding patients with stroke or mini-stroke, retinal vascular occlusion/ischemia, or nervous and musculoskeletal symptoms.

3. **Carotid endarterectomy** – Procedure to remove plaque build-up from a carotid (neck) artery in a patient to prevent stroke. Considered overuse when performed on female patients without stroke symptoms or a history of stroke.

4. **Coronary artery stenting** – Procedure to place a stent or balloon in a coronary artery. Defined as overuse when performed on patients with stable heart disease (not having a heart attack or unstable angina). Excluding patients with a past diagnosis of unstable angina.

5. **EEG for fainting** – A test of the electrical activity of the brain. Considered overuse for patients where syncope (fainting) is the primary diagnosis, and there is no history of syncope in the past two years.

6. **EEG for headache** – A test of the electrical activity of the brain. Defined as overuse for patients with a headache as the primary diagnosis on the claim and no history of headache in the past two

years. Excluding patients with epilepsy and recurrent seizures, convulsions, and abnormal involuntary movements.

7. **Head imaging for fainting** – Considered overuse for patients where syncope (fainting) is the primary diagnosis, and there is no history of syncope in the past two years. Excluding patients with epilepsy or convulsions, cerebrovascular diseases, head or face trauma, altered mental status, nervous and musculoskeletal system symptoms, and a history of stroke.

8. **Hysterectomy** – Procedure to remove the uterus. Considered overuse for patients without a diagnosis of cancer or carcinoma in situ.

9. **Inferior Vena Cava (IVC) filter** – Procedure to place a filter (a medical device) in the large vein in the abdomen to prevent blood clots from moving to the lungs. Considered overuse for all patients except those with a history of multiple pulmonary embolisms.

10. **Renal artery stenting** – Procedure to place a stent or balloon in the renal (kidney) artery. Considered overuse for patients with high blood pressure or plaque build-up in the artery. Excluding patients who had a diagnosis of fibromuscular dysplasia of the renal artery (abnormal twisting of the blood vessels).

11. **Spinal fusion/laminectomy** – Procedure to fuse vertebrae together (spinal fusion) or remove part of a vertebra (laminectomy). Defined as overuse for patients with low-back pain, excluding patients with radicular symptoms, herniated disk, radicular pain, or scoliosis; also excluding prior two occurrences within 30 days of radiculopathy, sciatica, or lumbago.

12. **Vertebroplasty** – Procedure to inject cement into the vertebrae to relieve pain from spinal fractures. Considered overuse for patients with spinal fractures caused by osteoporosis. Excluding patients with bone cancer, myeloma, or haemangioma.

TABLE: Examples of WaFEr frequently encountered in India:

1. Resorting to cesarean section delivery when a normal delivery is perfectly feasible.

2. Prescribing an expensive branded drug when a 10-fold cheaper generic equivalent is available.

3. Master health check-ups for the healthy (even when not so wealthy).

4. CT Scans and MRIs as a first-line diagnostic tool instead of careful history taking and physical examination.

5. Prescriptions padded with medicines of no value, e.g., multivitamins.

The Biomedical Arms Race: Proton beam treatment

In this century of accelerating biomedical innovation, we can look forward to life-changing and life-extending innovations of a wide variety. Some will be as simple as the Mediterranean Diet, which is of proven benefit. Others will be powerful new treatments with high efficacy like cell and gene therapy, where again the survival benefit is obvious. And then there is a third category of innovation where the technology is mind-blowing enough that despite the lack of robust evidence, it is put into practice.

Many of these innovations are in the area of diagnostics, where the regulatory regime is much more forgiving. Secondly, in a pure fee-for-service model where the incremental cost of any new device or treatment can be passed on easily to payers — the patient or his insurer — there is nothing to hold back an individual physician from resorting to the most recent glitzy technology, as long as it is not harmful. Finally, there is also medical arms race that for-profit hospitals are in. In a plain vanilla environment where hospitals try to differentiate themselves from the competition, high technology that is also expensive (and therefore affordable only by a few top hospitals) becomes the visiting card that hospitals use to attract patients. The equipment, even if not needed for most patients, still provides a halo of sophistication that the hospital can bask in. Once the top dog hospital starts advertising its high-tech equipment, then the competition also needs to invest in the equipment so as not to be seen as a laggard. The biomedical arms race is set in motion.

A recent example is proton beam therapy. Proton beam treatment has a higher tissue resolution compared to radiotherapy and is preferred for the treatment of some cancers in children or when there is an adjacent vital organ that needs to be protected[3]. The downside is that proton beam therapy is prohibitively expensive for widespread use. The average cost of entire proton therapy in cancer treatment would be between ₹ 25, 00,000 to ₹ 30, 00,000 (USD 33,000 to 39,000). As per a recent review - "The most secure estimate of percentage benefit (from proton beam therapy) was 4.3%, but insufficient clinical outcome data exist for confident estimates". Despite this, many oncologists have resorted to the use of PBT even in situations where there is no clinical evidence of its effectiveness over traditional radiotherapy. This is an example of a medical arms race, where the latest and glitziest is often conflated with being the best treatment.

In the UK, the National Institute of Clinical Excellence is charged with generating and using the evidence base from clinical trials to adjudicate on new technologies and their eligibility for use in the population under UHC. Unfortunately, such a mechanism does not exist in India. Unless we build this capability and deploy it soon, newfangled technologies that come at huge costs are likely to overrun any attempt at implementing UHC.

If costly treatments with doubtful utility get purchased by patients and their families who can afford to fund their treatment out of pocket, then can that be considered a benign waste? Not so for the following reasons:

(1) If you offer a treatment option with the thinnest marginal utility for a cancer patient who suffers from a terminal condition, then the tendency is for friends and family to step in and inject the resources

needed to purchase that treatment, especially if the treatment in question is hyped up as a last resort; parents may sell heirloom properties to fund treatment of a child in a last-ditch effort which may have the run on consequence of depriving necessities like a good education and healthcare for another child in the same family. The fact that the wealthy buy the treatment will signal to the rest that it is wise to follow suit, even if the costs are punishing. (2) If patients use their insurance to pay for treatments with marginal utility, then premiums will rise for everyone. (3) If the hospital providing this costly treatment incurs huge upfront fixed costs that are barely recoverable, then the temptation will be to subsidize the treatment by increasing costs elsewhere, thus making patients pay more for treatment that is essential in order to cover the costs for patients who are given treatments that are not necessary. Thus, costly treatments that provide marginal benefits are a waste and impose additional costs on the wider population, even when privately funded out-of-pocket by the rich. Wasteful absorption of resources by those who can afford it is not victimless.

Proton beam treatment exemplifies the new technologies that have the potential for overuse and misuse if left unregulated. But PBT is by no means a major drain on resources since it remains a rare intervention done at very few centers. Cesarean sections, on the other hand, are routinely done procedures in small nursing homes and big hospitals across the length and breadth of India. The patent overuse of cesarean sections to deliver babies is of greater concern, both immediately and in the long term.

03 | COULD THE PREFERENCE FOR CESAREANS SEED A RISE IN DIABETES?

Giving birth is a physiological process. Humans are at the terminal end of over 170 million years of mammalian evolution that has perfected the process of giving birth to live offspring. The baby enters the world through the vaginal passage. In obstetric parlance, this is called a 'normal' delivery, and it confers several benefits to both the baby and the mother.

Interfering with this process is fraught with downsides. However, for a variety of medical reasons relating to the fetus or the mother, a normal delivery is not always feasible. In such cases, the baby is extracted from the uterus using a surgical procedure called a cesarean section. This procedure has become safer under modern conditions, but that doesn't mean it is risk-free. A cesarean section increases the morbidity and mortality risk in the mother 4-5-fold relative to a normal delivery.

Despite the benefits of vaginal delivery, cesarean section rates are rising in many countries, and not in a way that is explained by medical factors alone. The data indicates that among patients who have medical insurance, cesarean rates are performed in 50% of all deliveries (this information is from a proprietary source available to one of the authors). But in public hospitals, where treatment is free, the cesarean section rate is much lower, at around 20%. At the premier Christian Medical College, Vellore, the rate is even lower, at around 15%[4]. One way to explain this disparity between hospitals is that the 'excess' cesarean sections may not be medically justified. According to the WHO, the cesarean section rate in a given population is expected to be 10-15% if the guidelines for prescribing a cesarean section are strictly followed.

The higher rates could be driven by considerations extraneous to the baby's or the mother's health. One of them is economic: Obstetricians are busy doctors and place a high premium on their time. A planned cesarean section takes around 30 minutes and can be scheduled at a convenient time. Normal vaginal delivery can take an indeterminate number of hours and can't be scheduled beforehand. A cesarean section could also earn a hospital up to 50% more than a normal delivery.

Add to this the anecdotal preference among many patients – especially of the insured class – to avoid pain. Some may also like to schedule the delivery for an auspicious time. Such factors come together to render a cesarean section more desirable. However, this calculus sidelines the medical needs of the mother and the baby.

Rates of C-Sections across countries and Indian states		
S.No	**Countries**	**Rates %**
1	China	47%
2	India	20%
3	USA	32%
4	Indonesia	19%
5	Mexico	52%
6	UK	29%
7	Bangladesh	35%
8	Nigeria	2%
9	Philippines	23%
10	Canada	28%
S.No	**States**	**Rates %**
1	Telengana	61%
2	Andhra Pradesh	42%
3	Kerala	42%
4	Jammu and Kashmir	42%
5	Goa	40%
S.No	**Across different settings**	**Rates %**
1	Government hospitals	16%
2	Private hospitals	30%
3	Private hospitals for insured persons	50%

We wouldn't have a problem if normal vaginal deliveries and cesarean sections resulted in similar clinical outcomes. But this isn't the case. Apart from the risk of an invasive surgical procedure due to excess bleeding, infection, and complications due to anesthesia[5], there are also longer-term consequences. For the mother, a cesarean section increases the risk of complications in subsequent deliveries[6]. For the baby, there is a well-documented increase in the risk of childhood obesity[7] and, to a lesser extent, asthma.

A 2020 study[8] published in the Journal of the American Medical Association showed a 46% higher risk of type 2 diabetes among women born of cesarean deliveries. Since type 2 diabetes itself increases the chance of having a cesarean section in the mother, the study's results indicate a sort of positive feedback loop that increases the need for cesarean sections with every subsequent generation of mothers. The authors of this study suggest a possible reason for their findings. When the baby is born via the vaginal route, it is exposed to bacteria in the birth canal. These bacteria colonize the baby's gut and may help regulate fat and glucose. The guts of babies born through cesarean sections are colonized by a less diverse population of environmental bacteria, which may not offer the same set or extent of benefits.

Data available for the US shows that cesarean rates have increased from 4.5% in 1965 to 32.2% in 2014. The corresponding prevalence of diabetes was lower than 2%; by 2014, it had increased to a little over 7%. With each generation of women, there will be a lag of 30–40 years between the time that they are birthed through a cesarean section and their diagnosis as diabetics. So the increased rate of cesareans in the 1990s is still to play itself out. And even if we stopped performing cesarean sections today, it could be another 30–40 years before we might see a change in the incidence of diabetes.

The link between diabetes and cesarean births calls for an urgent response at several levels. For starters, there should be a national mandate requiring hospitals to report their cesarean rates – coupled with a mandate for obstetricians to follow evidence-based guidelines to determine the need for a cesarean section.

Second, economic incentives that drive hospitals to prefer cesarean sections must be neutralized – for example, by equalizing the income from cesarean sections and normal deliveries.

The government should also consider reintroducing trained midwives to support obstetricians while attending to protracted 'normal' deliveries. The mother and her family must participate in the decision-making process. Many mothers prefer a cesarean section because they are afraid of the pain they have to endure during labor. However, fear alone shouldn't guide decision-making. They have to be counseled about the risks and benefits of their choice. This, in turn, will require a fully and formally documented informed consent process, using standardized educational materials.

The rising number of cesarean sections is ultimately a symptom of a wider problem. Wasteful and harmful medical choices driven by reasons other than patient considerations are generally common with costly procedures. In the US (for which the data is available), 50% of interventional procedures for coronary artery disease were found to be unnecessary or of uncertain benefit. Such unnecessary care diverts economic resources that could be applied to delivering healthcare for the poor.

Indeed, in the US, wasteful healthcare is believed to account for 25% of total healthcare costs. Using a similar estimate for India would imply the savings from avoiding unnecessary cesareans would be around Rs. 2,000 crore – with attendant benefits for health outcomes as well as the healthcare economy. A national body of experts constituted to include representatives from healthcare and insurance companies must be charged with examining this issue and implementing corrective measures. This can't be delayed without jeopardizing the health and economy of the country itself.

SECTION SUMMARY AND CONCLUSIONS

It is worth reminding ourselves of the following facts:

1. WaFEr can consume upwards of 47% of the healthcare budget; waste alone consumes roughly 20 to 25 percent of American healthcare spending. Excessive medical tests cost the US economy $200 billion. It is not the cost alone that is a problem; excessive testing can lead to false positive results that trigger further rounds of testing and sometimes even the wrong treatment.

2. It is not the absence of care, but care itself, that kills more Indians. - 1.6 million Indians died due to poor quality of care in 2016, nearly twice as many as due to non-utilization of healthcare services (838,000 persons).

3. The cost of a plain vanilla generic versus its brand equivalent can be as different as 10 to 20-fold. It is like paying 20 times more for salt when cheaper unbranded salt is available.

4. The cesarean rate, as per WHO norms, should be 15%. In Finland, it is 16.5%. In India, the rate at which cesareans are performed varies from 50% for privately insured patients to 15% for patients at CMC, Vellore (a private non-profit hospital).

5. Globally, 1.6 percent of annual deaths in children under 5 — more than 140,000 deaths — can be explained in part by corruption.

6. Around one in 20 patients is exposed to preventable harm during medical care.

7. There are at least 43 million injuries worldwide each year due to medical care, and nearly 23 million DALYs are lost as a consequence. A large majority of these injuries and harm occur in developing countries, and these numbers will likely grow.

In a world where healthcare costs are spiraling ever higher, it is foolish to allow WaFEr to compound the problem by consuming 50%

of healthcare expenditure. Tight public governance and transparency can go a long way in controlling WaFEr. The gatekeeper function of Comprehensive Primary Care can rein in runaway costs resulting from overuse of specialty care. For elective procedures, a negotiated fixed-price model can be used to control costs charged by service providers. Almost instantly, a move to strengthen the generics ecosystem and forcing providers to prescribe generics can take a huge chunk out of costs. Controlling WaFEr has to be done with urgency using all means available to us. This should include digitalization and automation to bring about transparency. Shining a light on the dark recesses of healthcare will unmask the unhealthy and unethical practices and force the changes that can effectively curb them.

HEALTH TECHNOLOGY

Health technologies should be the handmaidens for healthcare. Leveraging these technologies must be a key enabler for making UHC feasible - both from an economic and quality angle. This is also a place where India can shine as a world leader in innovation. But like everything related to healthcare, this needs policy direction and leadership from the Government.

While someday the computerization of medicine will surely be that long-awaited "disruptive innovation," today it's often just plain disruptive: of the doctor-patient relationship, of clinicians' professional interactions and workflow, and of the way we measure and try to improve things.

Robert Wachter, The Digital Doctor: Hope, Hype, and Harm at the Dawn of Medicine's Computer Age

The urban and rural tele-health demonstration projects of the 1970s did not fail because the technology did not work…. the programs failed to live beyond initial demonstration because there was neither professional endorsement, economic support, nor political will to build on the promise of telemedical systems.

Jeremy A. Greene in The Doctor Who Wasn't There (2022)

There is a "change layer" – the cloud in which visionary ideas about transforming healthcare reside. But there is also a "reality layer" – the place where most care is delivered. Both are necessary, but there is little mixing between them.

Sachin H Jain

..the barriers to a digital transformation in healthcare are often decidedly non-technological…

McKinsey Quarterly (June 2019)

The current allocation for healthcare in the Indian budget is about 2.4% of GDP. Including private expenditure on healthcare, the total spend is over 4% of GDP. If UHC becomes a reality, there will be a higher growth trajectory for healthcare expenditure (an example that is an outlier but a signal of the times to come is the cost of gene therapy, which can be over USD 3 million for a single patient's treatment). Given competing priorities that include non-negotiable elements like defense and education, it is clear that the increases in healthcare spending have to be managed carefully. One way to do this is to operate healthcare more efficiently, i.e. consume fewer resources to achieve the same objective.

There are a few levers the Government can use to manage the increase in healthcare spending. One is the near universal adoption of UHC; in a virtuous cycle, implementation of UHC can help control the loss of productivity due to chronic disease that can be added back as economic output available for spending on UHC. Another lever is to ruthlessly cut down on wasteful expenditure which can go unnoticed in healthcare, especially in tertiary healthcare, as discussed in the section on WaFEr. But there is a third lever that India can use to bring costs under control, and that is the appropriate use of technology. We use the term "technology" in the broadest sense to encompass both IT and non-IT technological solutions.

Three kinds of health technology

For this discussion, we can consider health technologies of three kinds. The first is the kind that may be expensive but significantly improves clinical outcomes when used appropriately. Costly imaging techniques like MRI, expensive new-generation cardiac stents, expensive diagnostic tests, and expensive new medicines all come under this category. While their appropriate and evidence-based use can provide significant clinical benefits, the same evidence can be used loosely as a justification for their unbridled application, even for conditions where they are not proven. Patients are only too willing to bear the costs. The supine insurance sector makes whimpering noises but is powerless to overrule decisions taken by medical "experts." The temptation for providers to overprescribe such income-generating interventions is irresistible.

The next kind of technology has clear benefits for the patient but is not associated with positive economic drivers of the kind mentioned above. Here, adoption is gradual but inevitable. Examples include health technologies that support frugal care for low-income patients or innovations developed for last-mile delivery of healthcare in remote regions. India is especially suited for the development and deployment of such technologies since the need is huge. An example is the FORUS ophthalmic exam system, developed by Bengaluru-based Forus Health - an ophthalmoscope that can be operated by a non-ophthalmologist, with interpretations of the captured images being offered via a cloud-based system. Given the shortage of ophthalmologists, especially in remote areas, this is an excellent first-line screening method that detects problems early. This is one of a family of affordable and robust healthcare devices and technologies that have been developed in India. Naturally, it is possible to build a use case for such a solution even in advanced economies, and FORUS is doing just that by entering markets outside India (in such markets, the cost arbitrage in terms of ophthalmologists sitting in India and reading the image can be a considerable advantage). This use of technology also has a benefit for doctors who can offer the screening service to their patients for a fee. So, a deserving technology also enjoys widespread adoption. Technologies like the FORUS ophthalmoscope, where there is both potential for increased income to the doctor and high benefit for the patient, will get adopted readily. These kinds of interventions are not displacing legacy investments, and because of their simplicity and low costs, they are the only option in environments where affordability is a barrier.

A third kind of technology is Health IT. Digitalization enables the automation of routine processes. Automation makes things convenient, faster, and cheaper. Automation can also eliminate errors that plague human-driven processes. Only thirty percent of tasks can be automated in healthcare, which is much lower than in other industries. But that is still a significant opportunity to reduce medical errors of the kind that cause serious injuries and cost lives. And yet, automation to a level that is commonplace in other industries is not seen in healthcare[1].

Digitalization in healthcare is work in progress.

Even something as simple as the Electronic Health Record (EHR; the equivalent of your online bank statement) is seeing implementation in fits and starts, with plenty of persuasion (Government grants in the US) and coercion (an NHS mandate in the UK) required to drive adoption. In India, the EHR is absent. It is not as if doctors are Luddites — their enthusiastic adoption of new drugs and medical technologies is proof. And yet, for clinical processes, the progress of digitalization has been glacial.

Digitalization is a problem for medical establishments. For one, it enables a high level of transparency and openness that can be threatening to players who are not playing strictly by the book. For example, a hospital that delivers inferior care resulting in frequent readmissions will easily be discovered. Furthermore, the extra effort and time taken to fill the information in these demanding electronic forms does not return a proportionate jump in income for the healthcare practitioner. EHRs were technologically feasible in the 1960s. Sixty years later, they are still far from attaining the ideal state of becoming a universally portable system of medical information. As Jeremy Greene says in his book "The doctor who wasn't" (2022) "the challenges reside in a gridlock of stakeholders… whose motivations point in several different directions." EHRs are often passively resisted and sometimes even actively resisted.

Commentaries on Health IT's failure to take root often point to the wrong examples. For instance, in an editorial in the periodical Modern

Healthcare, an example is provided of how Health IT is not doing its job. The author makes a comparison between a haircut and a doctor's appointment. Why, she asks, is it that we make an appointment with our hair stylist and expect it to be kept but when we make an appointment with a doctor we tolerate long waits before being seen? While long waits to see a doctor are an issue, they are less of a digitalization issue and more of a structural issue in the way healthcare is organized around the convenience of physicians. Digitalization has long been solving such problems in consumer industries like retail. But in medicine, the big bad problem is not waiting times; it is how can we improve clinical outcomes, how can we avoid killing patients by reducing medical errors, how can we avoid complications due to a botched procedure because someone did not use a checklist? These are the problems health IT should focus on. These are the problems where a solution will make a significant difference. Solving the "wait for the doctor" problem will not lead to a mad rush to adopt health IT. But saving lives by catching and preventing the mis-prescribing of drugs can force the adoption of a digital tool that does just that.

In the following section, we have four pieces: we start with a recap on why EHR adoption has been sluggish, and in "Slow to Tango," we provide solutions that can speed digitalization in healthcare. In the piece on Health Innovation Parks, we offer an architecture that can move healthcare innovations much faster through the pipeline in an ethical and regulated environment. In the piece on PrescribeNET, we offer a solution that can be easily deployed tomorrow all over India on the back of smart mobile phone platforms. Scalability is key, interoperability is key, and legislation and government mandates are enablers. The government should understand its indispensable role in making this happen, and fast-track these solutions.

02 | THE STUNTED EVOLUTION OF ELECTRONIC HEALTH RECORDS

Corporate hospitals, as early as the mid-80s, recognized the need for billing systems. This was also the time that India's IT sector was seeing its sunrise moment, and it was not uncommon for hospitals to hire IT professionals to build billing systems from scratch (Health Information Systems or HIS). Soon, hospitals recognized the need to go beyond billing, to front office automation and out-patient management, and in some cases inpatient management as well. Around this time, hospitals opted to outsource the development to IT services companies. Some like TCS, which had grown to a reasonable size (TCS revenues in 1990 were around Rs. 250 Cr), had a strategic interest in the Indian market for IT services and were preferred partners for hospitals moving their usage of IT to the next level.

In mature markets like the US, HIS companies develop products that they license to hospitals. Their implementation partners install the product, customizing it to hospitals' specific requirements. Customization efforts are priced high to dissuade needless customization. Unlike the HIS product companies in the US, the DNA of Indian IT services is different—most of their revenues come from building customized code in response to a specific set of requirements. To speed up this process, they might re-use some or all of the code they might have built-in earlier assignments. Indian IT services companies when were approached by hospitals to develop IT solutions for what hospitals perceived as unique requirements (a misplaced perception, since operating processes of most hospitals are similar), offered to customize the code they already had. However, the extent of customization asked for by each customer was so extensive that the product was not of much use to the next customer that came along.

Other issues played out in the Indian market as well. For example, widespread piracy led most users to believe it was foolish to pay for licenses. And since coding skills were available at low billing rates, hospitals were spoiled to expect customization at low prices. To keep their costs low, many providers of IT solutions adopted less than robust practices when building the solutions.

Market Development

In light of the multiple factors highlighted above, the Health Information Systems (HIS) business segment in India has underperformed. For comparison's sake, let us take the example of Cerner Corp, the largest HIS company in the US with $5.0 billion in revenues where the total healthcare sector is approximately $4.0 trillion. If there was an Indian Cerner with proportionate revenues we would expect that company to have revenues of around Rs. 1000 Crores. The reality is that there may not be a single HIS company in India with even 1/20th of that revenue.

Fragmentation in the HIS sector results in few clients for each HIS company. Combined with misplaced expectations from the hospital, it becomes extremely difficult to provide an appropriate level of technical support, thus adversely affecting the hospital's use of the IT solution. The resulting disenchantment drives hospitals to change service provider within 3-5 years. The HIS company loses clients as fast as it can acquire them. Hospitals also expect the new service provider to support them in porting data from their current system to the new one. This is easier said than done, and most hospitals end up with their data residing in silos in multiple systems. These are hardly ideal conditions for the growth of the sector.

Due to these reasons, despite hospital owners claiming total control over their data, their usage of their IT systems remains at a very basic level. There is a huge opportunity lost to make the data work for them to improve efficiency. With this kind of implementation, it is very difficult to demonstrate a respectable ROI on any level of investment in an IT solution.

Operational Constraints

Most HIS solutions available in India provide reasonable features to address hospital requirements for the front office, patient scheduling, billing (including third-party billing - health insurance, corporate relationships, etc.), pharmacy, radiology, and laboratory. However, even in these areas, the focus is on the financial and administrative aspects, with little attention being paid to the clinical aspects of patient care. Therefore, the large volume of clinical data generated during treatment - whether it is in the outpatient departments, operating rooms, or intensive care units - is still processed manually.

Getting Around the Constraints

The structure of the HIS market must transition from services to products. The key is for hospitals to recognize that their processes may not be as unique as they believe they are. Using off-the-shelf products will have the added advantage of expediting product selection and implementation. The consequent ability to improve utilization of HIS tools (supported by better product training) will deliver far better results and allow hospitals to realize a better return on their investment.

All it takes is for hospital owners to understand that their processes might be quite similar to (if not identical to) other hospitals of their size and type. If a particular department insists that a process needs to be customized, a cost-benefit analysis can quickly determine the value of such customization and help decide if it is needed. Efforts like this will enable hospital owners to approach their HIS investments rationally by linking them to expected outcomes.

On their part, HIS companies must also adopt the best practices of product companies. Foremost among which is to price customization efforts high, so that hospitals think hard before requesting minor customizations that have no or very little impact on outcomes.

In the next chapter, we diagnose the reasons for the "slow tango" between IT and healthcare. We also provide solutions applicable to a broader range of contexts apart from HIS.

03 | IT AND HEALTH CARE: A SLOW TANGO

Healthcare has made tremendous progress over the last one hundred years. Molecular therapies, imaging, transplantation, prosthetics, and implantable devices have made modern medicine a cornucopia of technological wonders. However, many of the processes and routines used today in the delivery of healthcare remain unchanged from a hundred years ago. The paper prescription is alive and thriving. We schedule appointments over the phone, and health records (if we keep them) are mostly papers in a file. Although the digital revolution has transformed other parts of the economy, the delivery of healthcare follows quaint rituals untouched by the transforming capabilities of IT. Your doctor still writes out your prescription in longhand, and you must be an obsessively organized filer if you can find your cholesterol level reports from two years ago. Even the Byzantine processes of the Income Tax department have been digitized. But healthcare's love for the fleeting paper trail remains strong.

Contrast this with your bank. They serve you through a spiffy online site, and it is rare to have a reason to visit the branch. If you do visit the branch, you do not have to bother carrying a passbook or papers of any kind; they have your financial history, including your credit score on the system, and can access all the information needed with a few mouse clicks.

Healthcare, with all its complexity, human touchpoints, and inconvenient process hand-offs, should be ripe for the adoption of digital tools. Digitalization enables the automation of routine processes. Automation makes things convenient, faster, and cheaper. Automation can also eliminate errors that plague human-driven processes. Only thirty percent of tasks can be automated in healthcare - much lower than in other industries. But that is still a significant opportunity to reduce medical errors of the kind that cause serious injuries and cost lives. And yet, automation of the kind that is commonplace in other industries is not seen in healthcare.

It is not as if digitalization cannot work in healthcare. Ninety-four percent of patients covered by the National Health Service in the UK have some kind of Electronic Health Record (EHR). But the NHS is a monolithic government-run system where coercion by fiat can prevail. In laissez-faire healthcare systems like in the US (which more closely resembles what we have in India), doctors had to be persuaded with financial subsidies to go electronic. In India, digitalization has not been mandated, and we muddle along with antiquated legacy systems.

The application of information technology to healthcare is especially relevant in India. We not only have to grapple with the healthcare needs of a large population, but we also have to do it with scant resources. Health IT enables the amplification of scarce resources to create scale. IT-enabled process improvements can enhance effectiveness and quality. The reduction of errors and elimination of waste, using IT tools, can be key to delivering healthcare on lean budgets.

As Indian healthcare companies and tech entrepreneurs explore innovative applications of tech to solve healthcare problems, they must answer the question -"Why is the adoption of tech in healthcare so slow?" If they knew the answer to this question, they could preemptively sidestep the implementation barriers they face. The stunning suddenness and scale of the COVID-19 pandemic highlighted the need for the massive deployment of IT in healthcare processes. Health-IT can be a key enabler that helps to achieve scale without compromising quality. The COVID-19 pandemic has accelerated technology adoption—an example is the sudden enthusiasm for tele-health by doctors. One hopes that when one citadel in healthcare falls to technology, the others will surely follow. But the path to full digitalization of health is not going to be a bed of roses unless health-IT entrepreneurs keep a mindful eye on the barriers along the way and find ways and means to overcome them.

Could the slow adoption of health-IT be a consequence of the reluctance of the medical profession to adopt new technologies?. The way hospitals are packed with glitzy technologies puts paid to this notion. Indeed, the medical profession often stands accused of an over-eager acceptance of new drugs and devices. So, what is it that makes the uptake of digital tools so slow in healthcare?

Resistance to change

Traditionally, medicine has been a conservative profession. Even when there is abundant evidence for the superiority of new treatments, doctors are reluctant to discard old practices for the new. This conservative attitude is reinforced by the Latin adage that all medical students are taught — primum non nocere — which translates roughly as "first, do no harm." In days when there were few effective treatments, a conservative culture made sense. It helped to rein in the temptation to try unproven snake oil remedies. However, this conservatism became a barrier when it came to proven and effective interventions. An early example of this was the resistance to handwashing before surgical procedures. In 1847 Dr. Ignaz Semmelweis showed the effectiveness of handwashing in reducing mortality from sepsis during childbirth. It took several decades before washing hands with soap became commonplace in medicine. A frustrated Dr. Semmelweis died in 1865 after suffering a nervous breakdown.

Doctors are eager beta testers for new technologies. Given the risk this may pose to patients, medical associations and regulators have in place very tight regulations. New technologies must run the gauntlet of regulatory barriers before being accepted. In the case of digital medicine, a key retardant has been the need to protect patient confidentiality. Since policymakers are not always conversant with the capabilities of new IT systems, they need to be convinced before allowing the adoption of a digital tool. Especially in countries like the US, any compromise in confidentiality can attract huge liability lawsuits. These circumstances have slowed experimentation with digital tools in healthcare.

Fragmented Ecosystem

There is a steep upfront cost to digitalization that low-cost providers are not willing to fund. Apart from this, the fragmented nature of healthcare delivery in India (the largest hospital chain Apollo operates less than 1% of all hospital beds in India) also retards the adoption of digital tools. Unless the entire ecosystem operates on the same standards and the digital documents are easily portable, the benefits are not fully available. If I visit Apollo Hospital today, and next month I visit Fortis, I cannot simply provide an electronic link to my Fortis doctor to access my past medical records. Electronic data, when it exists, does so in silos. This defeats the purpose of digitalization.

The isolated general practitioner, who should be the first point of contact for most patients, has limited ability to fund, maintain, and operate IT infrastructure, let alone a system that integrates with other specialists or hospitals to whom she refers patients. Healthcare is also fragmented across diagnostic laboratories, pharmacies, government and private hospitals, rehab centers, imaging centers, etc. These community-based centers are where patients receive most of their healthcare. There is a high level of stickiness in the relationship between patients and these service providers. This results in hyper-local oligopolies that actively resist changes that can dilute their control. For example, even if the hospital offers to create an access channel for the general practitioner for her patients admitted to the hospital, there is no incentive for the GP to use this channel to improve care coordination. Patients do not patronize doctors for the technologies they use. They patronize doctors with whom they have built a relationship. Since the doctor is a hyper-local monopoly she can be assured that the patient will report back to her clinic for the next illness' episode regardless of whether she offered IT-based care coordination support. Similarly, your neighborhood pharmacy has no incentive to offer an online ordering system, since online solutions dilute the value of the pharmacy's proximity to your home.

Furthermore, each component of the ecosystem has a divergent set of requirements, making a standard platform solution that operates across every component difficult to build. Even if such a platform were to be built, the question would arise as to who would pay to create and maintain such a system. This contrasts with the travel and airline industries, where the requirements are so uniform that a single platform can bring together a diverse set of service providers to provide services to customers.

Moral Hazard

Medicine is unique in splitting the role of payer (insurance company), provider (hospital), and consumer (patient). The payer is incentivized to control consumption, as opposed to the provider who is incentivized to increase consumption. Capping use of a service below what is needed or inflating use above what is required, are both not in the interest of patients. The misalignment of purpose between payer, provider and patient is compounded by an asymmetry of information. The consumer has no way of determining the appropriateness of the treatment prescribed. When there is a poor clinical outcome, the consumer has no way to know if this is due to poor quality treatment or simply bad luck.

As far as hospitals (providers) are concerned, a tech solution that increases revenues will get adopted fairly easily. A tech solution that decreases revenues, even if it makes a positive difference from a patient perspective, e.g., shorter wait times for appointments, will be resisted. The insurance company can also be expected to behave in its best economic self-interest. Unlike in the past, when individual doctors could be relied upon to use their best judgment to adopt innovations that benefit patients, the current corporate model of healthcare subjugates this motivation to the larger purpose of the corporate hospital to increase revenues and profitability.

A result is the slow adoption of EHRs Digitalization improves the efficiency of medical care - this is a benefit for the patient, in the form of convenience or improved clinical outcomes (because of fewer errors). For the Doctor, digital tools like EHRs are seen as an unwelcome imposition. It forces her to spend extra time completing the EHR without a corresponding increase in income. Digital records contain more information and can be stored, retrieved, and shared very easily, unlike paper records. This ease also means that digital records enable a level of transparency that paper records do not provide. This level of transparency can be uncomfortable for providers used to operating behind the guild-like opacity of traditional medical practice. While these factors may account for the smaller doctor-owned and operated facilities resisting digital tools, what accounts for the slow adoption of EHRs in professionally managed corporate hospitals, including Government-run hospitals?

Many "(mis)behaving" parts

Healthcare is complex. So is banking. But there is one crucial difference. The complexity of banking is in the multiplicity of transactions. However, each transaction is rule-based and can be mechanized to a point where an entry-level operator can use an automation tool. The nature of medicine and biology is that there are limited possibilities for automation. Care delivery in health calls for the orchestration of the action of a multiplicity of specialists - doctors, nurses, pharmacists, diagnostic technicians, insurance agents, etc., all of whom are highly trained professionals (and many of whom have the God complex!). The patient interacts one-on-one with this profusion of professionals to complete the circle of treatment, even for something as simple as surgery for a hernia. This sets up a new kind of complexity - the complexity of a system with many "(mis)behaving" parts. Healthcare professionals with their idiosyncratic behavior patterns, moods, and subjective biases add to the variability and complexity of medical transactions. For example, two doctors, seeing the very same patient, are unlikely to issue identical prescriptions. Which of them is right is not something machine intelligence is capable of arbitrating (as yet). You then have to make exceptions for variations in all parts of the healthcare delivery chain. At the diagnostic clinic, the phlebotomist may take 1 minute for a blood draw. But sometimes this can take 10 minutes. It depends on how prominent your veins are and how experienced the phlebotomist is. Such variations abound in medicine. It is impossible to automate human-variable processes using machine intelligence. The frequent allowances that have to be made for each anticipated exception will make the system so complex that it just does not make sense to automate.

The most important endpoint is least visible

In most businesses, say in a retail mall where tech is deployed, the value of tech to the customer is easily measured as customer delight. Many shops will ask you to choose between a smiley face and a frowny face at the checkout to record your overall satisfaction. And tech can be designed to improve the customer experience in very tangible ways. In healthcare, on the other hand, the most critical parameter is not so much customer satisfaction of the kind that retail businesses measure and treasure; the critical parameter that needs to be optimized is the clinical outcome. This is what patients should care the most about. But this is also the most difficult parameter to track, measure, report, and compare. If Hospital A has poorer clinical outcomes compared to Hospital B, it may simply be because Hospital A admits sicker patients. While many tech solutions will claim that they improve clinical outcomes, it is very hard to prove. The only things that are easy to prove are things like ease of appointment scheduling, reduction in wait times, speedy triage, and treatment initiation, etc. These parameters are only surrogate measures of how the outcome could be affected and may not accurately correlate with actual clinical outcomes. In a study of EHRs, the implementation of the EHR unexpectedly led to poorer clinical outcomes, since the distraction induced by the act of filling the EHR took time away from more important tasks like the physical examination and face-to-face interaction with the patient. The most important indicator of system performance—clinical outcome—that a tech solution should improve in a hospital is very difficult to track. And unless there is documented proof that clinical outcome is improved, a tech solution may be nice to have, but not essential. IT companies, therefore, are content with business models that deploy IT in a manner that there is an immediate and visible contribute to the bottom-line of the payer or provider. Blind-sided to clinical outcomes, such initiatives can boomerang by having deleterious effects on patient outcomes – it may be cheaper to discharge a patient from a hospital a day early, but not if early discharge results in a higher rate of recurrence and readmission.

Healthcare cannot be stormed by tech

If healthcare is idiosyncratic, so is tech, especially when done in start-up mode. The cultural baggage of tech makes it, in many ways, an unsuitable bedfellow for healthcare. Tech companies are often drunk on the Kool-Aid of Silicon Valley. They position themselves as mavericks, the barbarians at the gate, the archetype of the outsider. They operate alone. They operate in stealth. They make mistakes to learn from them. They put out unfinished prototypes and Trojan horses in the marketplace as the final product. They pivot 180 degrees overnight. They are not trustworthy partners who think of the long-term. They are cannibals who feast on the businesses of the competition; even the businesses of their partners. They do not seek incremental growth, they want exponential growth. They are disruptors-in-chief. They break to make. They do not care to study, understand and strictly comply with the regulations governing healthcare. Indeed, they will do everything possible to circumvent man-made constraints. In short, they are rich in qualities that do not fit very well with healthcare. This may be a somewhat exaggerated stereotype.

But at the start of the unfinished IT revolution in healthcare, it was certainly an articulation popularized by health IT executives.

Take the mission statement for Healtheon - "to use the power of computing and the internet to revolutionize the healthcare industry, stripping away its inefficiencies and inequities and streamlining it for the new millennium". We are well into the millennium and the "inefficiencies and inequities" remain, although Healtheon is long gone. Even more recently, the biggies — Google and Microsoft — have quickly retreated after seeing their initiatives, Google Health and MS Health Vault, fail to gain consumer traction.

The concept of 'disruption' does not sit well with healthcare. The healthcare system is complex with many large and entrenched players who would become instant losers if a "disruptive, alternative business model" came into play. Any change in clinical processes can also have unintended downstream consequences for clinical outcomes, and even if it does not, this argument will always be used by those resisting change to defend the status quo. In this battle of the Davids of IT versus the Goliath of Health, Goliath always wins.

Since Health Tech companies aspire to erase what exists and rebuild on the ruins, they do not put in the effort to understand what exists. Instead of chasing disruption, health IT companies would be better off deeply engaging with healthcare companies and doctors to find clear spaces and use cases where IT applications will find acceptance by the existing healthcare ecosystem. Yet another self-defeating tech start-up archetype is the tendency to operate alone, and in stealth. Healthcare innovation is better achieved by consortia of companies collaborating with each other and with the healthcare community to address problems. Tech solutions will find faster adoption if they integrate with existing business models. It is best to promote gradual change that gives room for entrenched players to adapt to change at a slower pace - "adaptive evolution" instead of "instant revolution". The disruption of the prevailing business model has to be more of an emergent property taking place over an extended period as the tech solution gets fully integrated and the opportunity for disruption presents itself as an easy segue.

Does this mean that the journey to digitalization in healthcare is going to be a protracted one? Not necessarily, if the Government played a lead role in smoothening the road. The HITECH Act (Healthcare and Information Technology for Economic and Clinical Health) was a piece of legislation the US Government used to drive digitalization. It cost USD 100 billion to implement in the form of incentives and generates 80 billion in annual savings. From a 10% EHR adoption rate in 2008, it has risen to 75%. It can be said that it succeeded, although a multiplicity of vendors pushing too many platforms and the resulting gaps in interoperability put paid to many of the high expectations. Such a carrot-and-stick policy can be adopted for India as well. In addition, simpler, more flexible, and modular designs for the tech solution will help to scale rapidly and facilitate interoperability. Interoperability is the golden grail for health IT. Interoperability ensures data liquidity that is essential for putting the data wherever it is held to multiple productive uses, including for the prototyping of new technologies. If we can achieve full interoperability, then the artificial walls that isolate data pools will be brought down. Healthcare providers will no longer have excuses for not providing patients with their data in a digital format.

The Government: Change Driver

Unlike economic activities in other sectors, most countries, even the most market-oriented economies, have the Government playing a key role as a change driver and regulator of healthcare. In India, especially as we move toward the avowed end-state of Universal Health Care, it is in the interest of the Government to enable healthcare delivery models that deliver quality healthcare for all citizens. The rapid absorption of digitalization in healthcare is a must if India has to scale such models at a cost that will not drown the national budget. Market forces alone will not be sufficient to make this happen. At the minimum, economic incentives provided by the Government must make this happen, as in the US. But even the US has been late and slow in the adoption of tools like the Electronic Health Record. In countries in Europe where there are strong national health systems, the adoption of EHRs has progressed much faster and can be an example of the path we must follow in India to enable rapid digitalization of health care.

The Indian Government has already laid out a vision for digitalizing healthcare, and this is contained in the National Digital Health Mission document. This is a fairly comprehensive approach that signals a strong intent. It is exactly the kind of top-down approach that can lead to a flourishing health-IT sector in India. But there will be many hurdles to cross before this national initiative can be rolled out. There are two aspects to this Government role that need close attention if the rollout must succeed.

Government has to be the rule maker and change enabler

Because of its sensitive and critical nature, healthcare can be a swamp for new technologies that have still not found a firm footing. The regulatory pathway puts stringent conditions for the introduction of new technologies in healthcare. Meeting these conditions strangles emerging tech solutions before they have seen the light of day. Displacing legacy systems that are not easily migrated to the new standard can also be an insuperable hurdle. These kinds of market barriers can only be lowered if there is a higher power that can arbitrate on standards and interoperability to ensure that innovations are not unfairly denied entry into the health tech marketplace. We need the playing field to be leveled to ensure fair competition and quick adoption of technologies that make a difference to clinical outcomes or improve the efficiency of the process, benefiting healthcare workers and patients. This is the role the Government must play.

Even free-market champions will concede the valuable role that the Government can play in healthcare. Government intervention that is proactive and preemptive has to set the guardrails within which competition and survival of the fittest can play out. A key role of the Government will be to set the standards. The VHS versus Beta-max standard type of conflict where the inferior VHS standard won simply due to the large installed base of VHS should not be permitted in healthcare, where the stakes are higher. Only best-in-class solutions must be left standing after the competition has played out. The Government cannot directly adjudicate between the two technologies. However the Government can ensure a level playing field for competing technologies to enable objective comparisons.

In a fragmented healthcare system, the only way to ensure the scalability of solutions and coordination of care for patients across the multiplicity of providers is the creation of mandatory interoperability standards for each piece of software that wants to plug into the system. The pieces that are plugged into the ecosystem can be created by innovative startups. By using the core interoperability standards, they will be able to compete as equals against larger players.

The introduction of tech in healthcare requires paying attention to other considerations that are specific to the nature of healthcare. This includes privacy standards and questions of who owns the data. These are also questions for which the Government should shepherd legislation and a rule-based environment (like TRAI for telecom or SEBI for the financial markets) that does not discriminate against smaller players. The Government has a key role to play, as an orchestrator and intermediary, using two powerful handles that only the government can use. The first handle is to establish standards for interoperability in cooperation with healthcare providers and IT companies. The second handle is to mandate universal adoption of these standards, perhaps by linking adoption to a licensing scheme for healthcare providers.

Shopping for healthcare

When we go to buy a consumer good, say a car, we have available to us an abundance of reviews by experts and comparative data on performance on which to base our purchasing decision. If you want the 0-100 KMPH measure of the car, you can get it. If you want to know how the car performed on the NCAP safety ratings, you can get it. You have the ARAI-determined mileage. Your car buying decision can be a highly informed one. Similarly, when you go to a healthcare provider, the least you want to know is how patients like you treated by a specific healthcare provider have fared in the past. Did they recover? How long did it take? How many suffered complications? How many came back within a month with problems? How long did they have to stay in the hospital? What did it cost? Now, if you had all these details for the 3 or 4 hospitals in your neighborhood, you can make an informed choice about which hospital to choose. The problem is that such data is seldom available. There are two reasons - hospitals do not want to share such information for obvious reasons, and even if they did, the data is not collected systematically to be made available in any useful way.

But the situation changes dramatically once we have EHRs Even if an individual's EHR is the confidential property of that individual, anonymized and aggregated data by hospital or by doctor can quickly be obtained. Indeed, the process of generating and analysing this data can be automated so that it is available for consumers to use in real-time.

For example, let us say you need an elective cardiac bypass, and you have to choose between hospital A and hospital B, then we can have the following kinds of data available:

1.   How many elective cardiac bypasses did each hospital perform

2.   How many days were the patients hospitalized

3.   How many required hospitalization within 3 months, 6 months, or 1 year

This kind of information, if made public, has two uses. One, it helps consumers make better choices. But, importantly, it also helps the laggards in the system to invest and work towards improving performance. And if they do not succeed in doing so, the customer will euthanize them with her feet. A virtuous cycle of improvement is set up that becomes unstoppable, with the customer playing a key role in determining who stays and who goes. The vital virtue of transparency can go viral once the consumer has experienced it.

In the next chapter, we suggest a means to get Health IT off the ground in India fairly quickly.

04 | A BIG YET SIMPLE IDEA TO GET TECH GOING IN HEALTHCARE

India faces massive challenges in the delivery of quality healthcare. Solutions to address this must be both simple and scalable to work in a country as large and complex as India. India has demonstrated the ability to leverage technology to successfully implement new initiatives on a massive scale, e.g., cashless online transactions (UPI) and biometric-linked identification (Aadhaar). What if we could do something similar in healthcare, specifically at the point where the rubber hits the road in the doctor-patient interaction—the prescription?

An estimated 4 billion prescriptions are issued by doctors in India each year. A majority do not conform to even the most basic quality standards as given by the WHO; common problems include unnecessary medicines and irrational (or even harmful) combinations of medicines. Handwritten prescriptions are often illegible and lack vital information about diagnosis and test results, making it hard to reconstruct the rationale behind the medicines prescribed. They are also prone to be misplaced, making it impossible to refer back and build a longitudinal history of the patient's illness. But what if prescriptions were generated and stored electronically? And what if electronic prescriptions could be sent to a permanent central store where they could be audited for quality? Could this be a first step toward moving healthcare toward an ideal state?

The technology to implement Electronic Prescriptions is mature; some 60% of prescriptions in the NHS (UK) are issued electronically. The software runs on smartphones, and the data can be easily transmitted using existing infrastructure.

Let us look at the workflow that can be built around PrescribeNET, a national electronic prescription infrastructure. Each prescription will have a unique electronic ID generated and issued on-demand by PrescribeNET. Demographic details on the prescription will be automatically captured from the unique patient ID assigned to every Indian citizen (which, like the PAN, can be linked to your Aadhaar). The electronic prescription will have all the necessary fields (with options for the doctor to customize as per the requirements of her practice), and any incomplete or wrongly entered fields will be automatically flagged so that the doctor can correct them. This includes warning flags for incompatible drugs or incorrect doses. Through the use of drop-down menus, manual text entry can be kept to a bare minimum, making the generation of the prescription easy and quick. Instead of handing over a piece of paper, the doctor's smartphone will automatically send a link that the patient can use at any time to retrieve the prescription from the PrescribeNET server. The patient will have exclusive control over who can access the prescription. The patient can share an electronic link to the prescription with the pharmacist to get the drugs dispensed. The information about the dispensing pharmacist and the batch number of the dispensed drug can be scanned and linked to the prescription, which now constitutes a complete record.

What this workflow enables is a 100% complete and model prescription. A near 0% error rate is achievable with a process that automatically flags errors. If doctors do not self-correct these errors (for example, prescribing antibiotics when not required), then the real-time scanning of incoming prescriptions by AI tools running on the PrescribeNET server will flag such occurrences and trigger warnings, additional training, or disciplinary action, as required.

Additional benefits can be derived from PrescribeNET. The National Center for Disease Control can set up auto-alerts to flag any unusual prescription trends suggestive of emerging epidemics. For example, a sudden surge in prescriptions for antibiotics will trigger an alert and an investigation. A localized spurt in cancer cases can be investigated for possible local carcinogenic causes, like environmental contamination.

Since batch numbers of drugs prescribed are available, the data can be used to alert the regulator to drug failures resulting from problems in the manufacture or counterfeit drugs. When new drugs are introduced, the regulator will be able to keep an eye on emergent issues relating to drug toxicity and side effects. The relative efficacy of drugs for a specific disease can also be studied. The huge wealth of data can be analyzed and insights used to spur innovation.

Electronic prescribing tools are already available. They are usually sold to doctors as a component of a complete EHR solution. And as always, interoperability issues are left unaddressed since we do not have a national body regulating and enforcing standards. The vision for PrescribeNET is a nationally mandated system, more like the PAN number we use to tag financial transactions. Using your PAN number, every major financial transaction an individual has participated in can be traced. PrescribeNET will do the same for the prescription – the healthcare equivalent of a financial transaction. The only difference will be that the control of the contents will rest with individuals, although anonymized content will be accessible to regulators.

The cost of implementing such a system nationwide (in remote parts of the country, there may be an interim paper-based system) will be more than compensated for by costs saved by avoiding needless, irrational, and harmful medicines. Indian skill sets in IT, specifically AI and Blockchain Technology, can be applied to make this a world-class system that eventually morphs into a more comprehensive electronic health record for every citizen. Electronic prescriptions can also be prototyped and tested in the Health Innovation Parks described in the next chapter.

05 | HEALTH INNOVATION PARKS: A SLINGSHOT FOR HEALTH TECH

We have commented already on the relatively slow penetration and slow adoption of technology (we are talking mainly about IT here) in healthcare. This is partly due to regulatory barriers and partly due to the complexity inherent to healthcare. If technology has to penetrate healthcare, then a protected sandbox for prototyping new products is necessary. The government should create these sandboxes by earmarking premier government healthcare institutions, like the AIIMS institutions, as places where controlled experimentation on new health tech innovations can be undertaken. The sandbox environment should have a soup-to-nuts approach to facilitate each step of the innovation process. The model we propose below has the potential to make India a world-beating leader in the development and deployment of technology solutions in healthcare.

As we have highlighted earlier the development, dissemination, and large-scale adoption of health tech have been hampered by (1) the lack of standards, resulting in a fragmented marketplace, (2) low and slow adoption by healthcare providers, who are reluctant to replace legacy systems and processes, (3) Ethical and regulatory issues that surround the development of healthcare innovations that directly impact the lives and privacy of consumers, (4) A tragedy of the commons, since the benefits of health tech implementation largely accrues to the Government and consumers, and not to private players.

Health, and by inference the health tech sector, is like telecom where the Government has a key regulatory role to play. But beyond the role of the Government as a rule-maker, we also envisage a key role for the Government as coordinator and catalyst for health tech innovation. The Government can level the playing field for innovation creating scope for competitive forces to ensure that the best solutions are curated, keeping the interests of healthcare consumers in mind.

We propose an innovation model that has the potential to make India a leader in the development and commercialization of health tech globally. Such leadership will not only benefit Indian patients and the Indian economy but can also become a huge export industry that combines products and services. The model we propose will, in one stroke, eliminate the common barriers that retard the development of health technologies as mentioned above.

The core of the model we propose consists of what we call Health-tech Innovation Parks (HIPs). These Innovation Parks will co-localize, both physically and organizationally, health tech companies, hospitals, clinics, mobile- and tele-health providers, regulatory agencies (IT, Health IT, Healthcare), medical research organizations, medical training/teaching institutes (like the AIIMS), ethics bodies, and the Clinical Trials regulator, Start-up companies, Investors, and International Collaborators. These parks will be safe spaces where new technologies can be deployed under controlled conditions, in compliance with the regulations that govern their experimental prototyping and testing. Such studies will be monitored, and the outcomes evaluated by independent experts who will evolve standards that can help in the progressive development of technologies. The process will ensure the development of technological solutions optimized for scalability. There is room for more than one HIP, with each HIP leveraging the strengths of local regions and specializing in specific technological domains, e.g. medical devices or robotics or AI/ML.

The innovation process in the HIPs should incorporate the methodology of design thinking. Design thinking prioritizes deep empathy for end-user desires, needs, and challenges to fully understand a problem. Such an approach helps develop comprehensive and effective solutions. Empathetic engagement with patients and their needs is the starting point. Two other elements of the design thinking process as applied to healthcare are radical collaboration and rapid prototyping. Radical collaboration recognizes the fact that "health problems exist across and at the intersections of disciplines and sectors, not within them". Patients, nurses, doctors, engineers, automation specialists, managers, technicians, and product development specialists have to collaborate to come up with robust and practical solutions. Design thinking also mandates "rapid prototyping". The advantage of combining "rapid prototyping" with "radical collaboration" is the opportunity to test prototypes across diverse stakeholders and get real-world insights that can help design solutions that work in the real world and not just in the laboratory.

Quoting from a paper by Roberts and colleagues (2016)[2]: "Much of the skepticism and frustration linked to the scale and pace of change and innovation within the current health system stems not from a lack of vision, effort, or even resources; rather it arises from attempts to remake a healthcare model never designed to do the things now being asked of it. We argue that expanded capacity for and application of design thinking approaches within healthcare can help drive necessary innovation in care delivery models. There is no single 'right' or easy answer to the challenges healthcare faces now and in the future, but the design thinking framework offers an accessible and recognizable approach for discovering, developing, and delivering services (both old and new) that align with individual and community needs".

Since design thinking would need co-location of the designers with the users (patients and HCWs), the HIP would provide the optimal conditions and locations to offer a tightly iterative process of do-learn-do that can produce superior solutions than those that are developed using more loosely integrated innovation practices. If the HIP is the Y-shaped wooden piece in a slingshot, then design thinking can be imagined as the elastic band that launches the missile (innovations) into action.

Health Innovation Parks can have a broad scope, offering a test bed for new health technologies, ranging from pure IT solutions to automation solutions/robotics and medical technologies. HIPs and the companies that run projects in the HIPs can be provided loans, tax incentives, and other privileges during the development phase. HIPs can invite partnerships with countries like Singapore, which do not have the population size needed for the rapid testing of new technologies.

CASE EXAMPLE: Tele-health

Tele-health has the potential to revolutionize how healthcare is delivered. It is especially important for India with its vast and dispersed population, where large swathes of the country suffer from inadequate healthcare facilities. For the development of tele-health, we need three ingredients: (A) Technology development; (B) Standards (including interoperability and electronic record integration standards); (C) A test bed where tele-health technologies can be rapidly prototyped under ethical and medical oversight.

Item (A) above is rapidly developing in the country, especially in the startup sector. However, these companies are hampered by the absence of an ecosystem that dynamically allocates resources to the best ideas with assurance that the fully matured product will be scalable across the country. The Government through its digital health mission is empowered to set the Standards – (B) above. What is needed in order to catalytically nurture and grow innovation in this area is to provide an environment where competing technologies can be prototyped and evaluated by technical and medical experts under a design thinking prototyping framework provided by a Standard-setting regulatory authority. If the HIP can co-localize an AIIMS with the companies developing the technologies along with model healthcare networks (from AIIMS to Primary Healthcare Centers) where the technologies can be evaluated, the speed of developing best-in-class solutions will be accelerated manifold. India, with its large technical manpower, medical expertise, and patient load, is well placed to become a world power in the rapid, cost-effective development of highly scalable health tech solutions.

For the Government, a single ministry needs to be tasked with this objective. Unfortunately, health tech falls in the gray zone between ministries. Since the subject has inter-ministerial ramifications, and hence may not be owned in all its scope by a single ministry, it may be best to form a cross-ministerial task force entrusted with the implementation of the Health Innovation Parks.

SECTION SUMMARY AND CONCLUSIONS

The following fact alone is enough to show how far behind we are in the healthcare technology space:

95% of prescriptions in the UK are electronic. Less than 1% of prescriptions in India are electronic.

The application of information technology to healthcare is especially relevant in India. We not only have to grapple with the healthcare needs of a large population, but we also have to do it with scant resources. IT enables the amplification of scarce resources to create scale. IT-enabled process improvements can enhance effectiveness and quality. The reduction of errors and elimination of waste, using IT tools, can be key to delivering healthcare on lean budgets. Translation of tech innovation in healthcare is, therefore, of the greatest importance.

Despite India's very high rate of adoption of digital systems in the financial sector, the healthcare sector has remained a laggard. The reasons are not far to seek: lack of uniform standards for interoperability, vested interests that fear the transparency that will arise from the digitalization of healthcare, and a lack of understanding of the many favorable roll-on effects of healthcare digitalization, including improved clinical outcomes.

The cultural norms that guide the behavior of information technology companies as disruptors may not work in healthcare. Health tech companies must be prepared to collaborate with a variety of stakeholders, including other startups that operate in adjacent areas. The preferred choice for tech deployment in the early stages should be to adopt business models that do not pose an existential threat to existing players, especially doctors. Doctors should be a part of the strategy team in health tech companies. Healthcare workers, doctors included, are often seen simply as consumers of technology. Health tech leaders need to move on from this perception and co-opt doctors in the technology development process since they understand best the peculiarities of medicine as it is practiced and will be able to point out gaps that may not be perceived by technopreneurs.

With the volume of patients we have, combined with our tech talent, India can become a leader in streamlining healthcare using judicious deployment of tech interventions. As long as the clinical outcome and comfort of the patient are always borne in mind, this explosion of innovation can lead to a thriving health tech sector. We have been waiting too long for that to happen. Perhaps the learnings and experiences from the COVID-19 pandemic will be used by the government to earnestly set the ball rolling on the digitalization of healthcare.

Until recently, the government has stood back from its role in developing the digital economy in the healthcare sector, under the facile but wrong assumption that leaving it to private players in the market as in other parts of the economy would work. Enlightened government oversight may be an oxymoron, but it is the only way to succeed in developing a coordinated approach that can nurture and grow this sector.

Healthcare is unlike other parts of the economy, where market forces can be relied upon to select winners. Healthcare is also where digitalization is sorely needed. Far from being an albatross around the neck of healthcare, health technology can be the wings taking Indian healthcare to the heights of performance and excellence it is capable of. The implementation of 5G and 6G technologies in many countries will accelerate the development of tele-health and robotics. India has the strengths to be a player in this field. India can also lead the field if we choose to deploy policies that facilitate the development of these technologies. A proactive approach led by the government is the only way that the digitalization of healthcare can proceed.

MISSION POSSIBLE

Universal Health Coverage is an imperative if we are to succeed as a nation. We show how UHC is eminently doable in India.

…(every) family had access to needed medical care, made possible and available to all Germans, rich or poor, by the social insurance system German chancellor Otto von Bismarck established in 1883. Germans may not always have had enough food in those years, but all had the health care they needed.

– From the book Priced Out, by Uwe Reinhardt

We feel that a nation's health is perhaps the most potent single factor in determining the character and extent of its development and progress. Expenditure of money and effort on improving the nation's health is a gilt-edged investment which will yield not deferred dividends to be collected years later, but immediate and steady returns in substantially increased productive capacity.

– Bhore Committee Report

What we face, is above all a moral issue; at stake are not just the details of policy, but fundamental principles of social justice and the character of our country.

– Ted Kennedy, in a note to President Obama, written just before he died, in the context of Obama trying to get the Affordable Care Act passed.

Health inequalities do not arise as a system of economic production behaving in unfair and illogical ways but as a system working in the only way it can, through the process of exploitation at its center, which is thoroughly injurious to human health.

– Lee Humber in his book Vital Signs

01 | PAYING THE PIPER

In this section, we address two related issues. The first is: What model of Universal Health Coverage is a feasible objective given competing priorities in a developing economy like India with vast inequalities in wealth, and a significant proportion of the population living in poverty? We argue that poverty and health are interrelated, and addressing health equity will also address some of the pernicious inequality. The second question is: Should this be on the back of a privatized corporate service model that is increasingly dominating the healthcare landscape in India, or do we need a new model that, while taming and corralling private for-profit efforts, does not eliminate them but allows them to coexist with a rules-based government-regulated ecosystem?

A healthy population generates wealth

It is understandable that economic growth will generate surpluses that governments can invest in the improvement of the health of their citizens. But the converse is also true. Better health can also improve economic output. How? As per the economists David Bloom and David Canning (1999)[1], improved health increases labor force productivity and therefore increases income. Healthier citizens are also motivated to invest in their education and skills since they can recoup the costs over a longer working life. Workers who know they are going to live longer also save for retirement, creating a pool of capital that is available for building physical infrastructure that benefits the economy. Finally, a reduction in fertility due to a reduction in infant mortality shifts a larger proportion of the population into the working age bracket, thus increasing productivity at the aggregate level in the medium term (the demographic dividend that is observed in developing economies). They estimate that a 5-year improvement in life expectancy can lead to a 0.3 to 0.5% faster growth rate, which can be a substantial boost to the economy. For India, this could be an addition of US $ 1750 Billion to the GDP in 2050 (almost 15% higher than the projected US $ 13.1 Trillion).

There are a few contentious points we would like to get out of the way. One is the role of private for-profit healthcare in a system of UHC. Our position is that laissez-faire for-profit healthcare is not desirable. For-profit healthcare has a corrosive effect due to the unnatural segregation of interests and the resulting creation of perverse incentives to increase the volume of care without caring about appropriateness and quality. What do we mean? Simply put, asymmetry of information and lack of immediate signals of quality assessable by a consumer means that typical market forces do not operate to discipline the greed of for-profit players. We need a payment system that guardrails the system to prevent the excesses of an untrammeled for-profit system.

If there is a large enough market of wealthy people willing to pay usurious prices for healthcare, then providers will gravitate to that end of the market and provide them with all the bells and whistles that they think they need. This is the situation in India now. Newly minted millionaires are driving prices up at the high end of the market. This trend is visible in the real estate market where prices at the high end have reached stratospheric levels. When this happens in healthcare, the low-margin business of providing care to low-income consumers is vacated by premium players who are then replaced by unorganized small-time providers without the infrastructure or systems to provide the complex treatments needed for diseases like cancer.

For-profit providers can deliver healthcare at an affordable price point, as long as incentives are designed to reward them for doing that. What we need is what has been called 'managed competition'[2]. Managed competition is a mechanism whereby costs are contained in a for-profit marketplace by fostering competition between providers of contracted services. Large buyers, such as the Government, can have healthcare providers bid for bulk contracts for providing healthcare services – say a contract to provide all the elective cardiac services in a given region with an ensured minimum volume.

A hybrid system that combines the efficiency of private players and the accountability of public systems is ideal. A backbone of public systems can drive both accountability and efficiency through a system of managed competition in which discretionary and emergency healthcare service delivery ("solution shops") is provided through publicly owned or controlled facilities, while the delivery of services that can be standardized, e.g. elective surgery, is contracted to private players (operating "focused healthcare facilities") who compete against each other based on both cost and clinical outcomes.

To foster meaningful competition, the playing field must be level. One player cannot be penalized because the mix of patients they see need more complex and expensive treatment compared to patients seen by the competition. There are two options to circumvent this problem: the first is to farm out to private contractors those pieces of healthcare that (on the aggregate) have high predictability of costs and outcomes, e.g., elective surgical procedures. Private contractors can operate efficient focused care facilities where elective procedures are done at high volumes. Incidentally, a high volume of procedures of the same or similar kind, for example, joint replacement, will also automatically improve the quality of work, as we saw in the first section. The second option is for a private player to manage a healthcare facility by charging a fixed management fee, similar to what hotel brands do with property owners, with an upside for delivering better clinical outcomes at a lower cost.

Single-payer versus multiple-payer systems

What kind of payment system at the level of the individual healthcare consumer works best? The simplest system is a taxpayer-funded system that is free for all comers for all treatments provided through a state-run system like the NHS. In many ways, this is an attractive option since it eliminates administrative overheads of managing billing, payments and insurance claims processing, etc. The downside is moral hazard—smokers and non-smokers are treated alike in the system, although the former group costs taxpayers a lot more money. Furthermore, government-owned and run systems have no incentive to improve efficiency and cost-effectiveness.

On the other hand, we have the example of the US, which has a multi-payer insurance system that expanded enormously after the Second World War. While this has brought a semblance of order to the system, it has also increased complexity, administrative costs, and the exquisite ploys insurance companies deploy to deny insurance. Today, US healthcare is in a crisis that is reflected in the poorest health outcomes among OECD countries at the highest cost. Multi-payer insurance systems where the ball can be kicked around between a forest of payment mechanisms have not provided a sustainable solution. It has merely lengthened the fuse toward the ultimate implosion of the system.

In this section, we reject payer models at both extremes—the taxpayer-underwritten model of the UK-NHS and the corporate model that is increasingly fertile ground for private equity. We propose alternate models that meld the best of both worlds—the efficiency-driven approach of the for-profit private sector and the patient and society-centric approach of the public sector.

Payment Models Currently Used

As per the National Health Accounts Estimate for 2018-19, the most recent compilation of data released in Sep 2022, health insurance (including all social health insurance programs) accounted for under 10% of all healthcare spending. So clearly, over 90% of all healthcare spending is from sources other than health insurance.

In this essay, we delve into the details of how Indians pay for healthcare services and provide comparisons to other countries.

Tax-funded Healthcare

India has numerous government-owned healthcare facilities (hospitals, health centers, dispensaries, etc.) where healthcare is free for the user. This is paid for from the budgetary allocation made by the government from tax payer funds. This method of paying for healthcare services is a key component in the current scenario, accounting for close to 25% of total healthcare spending. In countries where the government is the dominant provider of healthcare services like the UK, Germany, and Japan, tax-funded healthcare could account for over 75% of the total, whereas in countries where healthcare is split between the government and private sectors, it is around 50%. Tax-funded healthcare is usually comprehensive and provides access to outpatient and inpatient care and includes diagnostics, treatment, and medicine supply, without any caps on the quantum of care consumed. Services are provided through facilities owned by the government, which could be the central or state governments, and in many instances urban or rural local bodies.

Employer-paid Healthcare and Health Insurance

In some instances, healthcare expenses are paid by employers, both from the government and private sectors, for serving employees, and in some cases for retirees, as well as eligible dependents. Payments are typically made by the employer directly to empanelled providers from a fund set up for this purpose and administered in-house or outsourced to a third-party administrator. Most government departments like the defense and central government offices, as well as public sector enterprises, adopt this practice which at one time was quite prevalent even among private sector companies. This practice is referred to (perhaps inappropriately) as self-funded health insurance. Currently, this accounts for slightly over 8% of all healthcare expenses. Employer-paid healthcare is comprehensive, provides access to outpatient and inpatient care, includes diagnostics and treatment, and tends not to be capped. In the US, for instance, employer-paid healthcare accounts for more than 90% of total spending.

Starting in the early 2000s, employers saw in health insurance an opportunity to expand their employee benefits cost-effectively, and this segment took off exponentially with annualized growth rates of ~ 40%. A typical employer-sponsored health insurance policy provides coverage up to a certain amount (the sum insured, the median amount currently being in the ballpark of INR two lakhs) for inpatient treatment to the employee and dependents, which could include a spouse, children, and in many instances, parents as well. The entire premium amount might be paid by the employer, or the employee might be required to pay some part of the premium. Over 100 million employees (and dependents) of private companies receive this benefit, yet this accounts for under 5% of the total healthcare spending. The key difference between tax-funded and employer-paid healthcare and employer-sponsored health insurance is the absence of a sum insured or upper limit on spending in the former. Health insurers underwriting employer-sponsored policies tend to include risk mitigation features like sub-limits and ailment caps, and features like waiting periods and exclusion of pre-existing disease coverage are dispensed with.

Government-sponsored Social Health Insurance

Insurance has now become the preferred route for the delivery of healthcare even for the government, and many social health insurance schemes have been launched to benefit citizens at the bottom of the pyramid. The Ayushman Bharat program now seeks to subsume all these into one countrywide program, with minor state-wide variations. Health insurance has tended to pay only for inpatient treatment, diagnostics, and medicine supplies related to inpatient treatment. More importantly, health insurers may specify an upper limit (to the sum insured) and also incorporate sub-limits, as well as caps on specific treatments to manage risk.

Government-sponsored social health insurance schemes have expanded to cover over 300 million beneficiaries from the bottom of the pyramid. These schemes have evolved over the years and provide fairly extensive coverage (the sum insured is up to Rs. 5.0 lakh). For inpatient treatments that may not be available at government-owned facilities, these schemes provide access to private hospitals. For care that is not covered by the scheme individuals have to necessarily depend on Government hospitals and clinics. Government hospitals have been encouraged to expand their range of services and compete for patients with private hospitals. These schemes free up the supply side, but the absence of checks on quality and performance means that outcomes may not justify the costs.

Self-purchased Health Insurance

For a long time, most private health insurance was employer-provided. In recent years, individuals have started purchasing health insurance on their own, though very often it is to supplement employer-provided benefits. Today, over 50 million individuals own a health insurance policy purchased directly by them. These policies tend to resemble the group medical cover purchased by employers for their employees but will include features like waiting periods and exclusion of pre-existing disease. These policies will pay only for inpatient treatment in a hospital up to the sum insured. The sum insured can be enhanced through top-up or high-deductible policies, where the policyholder agrees to pay up to a certain amount, called the deductible or defined amount, after which insurance benefits kick in. Historically, self-purchased health insurance's share of health expenses has been lower than that for employer-sponsored health insurance (but only by 15-20%), but after a period when the gap with employer insurance was on the rise, it appears like the gap is narrowing, and it will not be surprising if self-purchased insurance was to assume a larger share within the next few years, mainly on account of two reasons: one, higher awareness results in an increase in self-purchased insurance, and two, employers no longer find health insurance to be a cost-effective employee benefit.

Out of Pocket Expenditure

In the end, all healthcare expenses have to be paid for, whether by the government (as a tax collector, as an employer, or as a sponsor), the employer (either directly or through health insurance), or the individual (through insurance or directly from their own sources of funds). In all scenarios except when individuals pay directly there are two balancing factors that come into play: risk pooling and oversight against fraud and abuse. These checks and balances are not present when an individual pays directly (out of pocket or OOP), which is what makes the high share of OOP a matter of concern. Sometimes, out-of-pocket spending does not come from an individual's own sources of funds, but from borrowings (from family and friends, and often from informal lending sources) or the sale/mortgage of assets, which is of greater concern because it has the potential to push individuals and families into a debt trap and poverty.

From close to 70% of all health spending coming from OOP in 2013-14, the share of OOP came down to 50% in 2018-19, even though the absolute amount was almost the same. After a steady annual increase until 2017-18, the OOP figure seems to be coming down, and hopefully the increase in government tax-funded spending and all forms of third-party payments will help bring down not just the share of OOP but the absolute amount as well.

Is there a right way to pay for healthcare?

The per-capita spend on healthcare is in the ballpark of Rs. 4000 per year. That would hardly be a stretch for even the lower-income group. Unfortunately, healthcare expenses rarely occur at the average level. Most of us will easily get by with a couple of visits to a doctor during the year, with maybe a few tests thrown in and some medicines, with a total cost much lower than Rs. 4000. Even those with limited means could easily receive the required treatment at a nearby government facility without incurring any costs. However, an unlucky few could end up with medical treatments that might not be available at the nearby government facility, requiring them to travel significant distances to a government facility or pay beyond their means at a nearby private hospital. Or they might require costly treatment that could strain the finances even of the relatively better-off. The table below summarizes cost of treatment data from the NSS 75th Round report (2017-18)

S.No	Category of spending (per event)	Treatment location	Approx Cost (Rs)
1	Outpatient care	Government facility	350
		Private facility	1100
2	Hospitalization	Government facility	4500
		Private facility	32000
3	Childbirth	Government facility	2700
		Private facility	24000

So, what is the right way to pay for healthcare?

The most commonly used healthcare service is primary care. Preventive care is also delivered through primary care via interventions like screening and annual health check-ups. In a system of UHC, primary care also has a gatekeeper function that determines when referral to secondary and tertiary care is needed. For these reasons, primary care should be made entirely friction-less. One way to make it friction-less is to make it universally free.

However, any public good that is completely free has a tendency to be overused. There is also a moral hazard with some citizens not taking health precautions in the knowledge that free healthcare is available. Therefore, it is appropriate to have a co-pay system where each encounter is partially paid for by the patient.

How do we ensure that primary care is available even to those who cannot afford the co-pay? A mechanism to do this is to credit every citizen with a fixed amount of "health credits" each year. The "health credit" can be linked to the UPI account and can be exchangeable exclusively as co-pay for healthcare services. Every 3 years, a proportion of health credits can be made encashable so that citizens are incentivized not to overuse the health credits they receive.

For example, if you receive 1000 health credits, 100 may be compulsorily allocated for annual health check-ups—these will not be transferable to other health services or become encashable. The remaining 900 can be used to co-pay for health encounters in primary care. If only 300 are used in a year, the balance will get carried over to the following year for 3 years in a row. At the end of 3 years, 50% of the balance of health credits (apart from the 100 allocated for annual check-ups) will become encashable. Encashability can be provided as an option only if the annual check-up has been availed of.

Such a system can ensure appropriate use of primary healthcare, including prevention-oriented services. But what about secondary and tertiary care? The costs in secondary and tertiary care are incurred as spikes that do not happen every year or with any regularity. There are also significant quality, efficiency, and choice of provider issues that need to be handled if we have private providers in the mix. This may be more amenable to payment through insurance. Those who cannot afford it will have their insurance premium paid through a government scheme. Both Government and Private insurers can be in the fray, competing for this business. While all citizens will have access to the no-frills insurance scheme, those who desire should have the option, for an additional premium, to access luxury services such as single rooms, without any change in the quality of essential clinical care which should be uniform for all.

Those who can afford it will also have the option of stepping outside the above choices (except for primary care, which should be mandated and compulsory, whether used or not) and access healthcare privately either for cash or through concierge care paid for through private insurance.

Whether we should spend 2% or 7% of our GDP on healthcare is the wrong question to ask. The right question is: What do we need to spend to achieve the population health outcomes we seek?

The national budget for 2023 is out and has allocated 86,000 Crs for healthcare. Adding in estimates for state budget allocations and out-of-pocket expenditure, the allocation for healthcare as a percentage of GDP rises to over 2.5%. The fraction of GDP that India's allocation represents compared to what other countries spend on healthcare is relatively small and a cause for public concern. For example, OECD countries spend around 7% of GDP on healthcare, and so does China. The predictable knee-jerk reaction to this is - "we should spend more on healthcare." But, should we simply spend more money on healthcare?

The relationship between expenditure on healthcare and health outcomes is not linear. The US, which spends the most on healthcare (18% of GDP), should have the best healthcare outcomes but it does not. In a fee-for-service system, an increased volume of care translates to higher profits for providers. In such a system, hiking cash allocation to healthcare will drive the prescription of unnecessary care, with adverse consequences for patient health. To avoid oversupply-driven inflation of demand, supply has to be tailored precisely to match the actual need.

So, how do we tailor the budget to match the requirements? First, we need to get out of the mindset of setting targets that are a fraction of GDP. It is not whether we spend 0.5% of GDP, 5% of GDP, or 15% of GDP on healthcare that matters. The "How much?" question has to be secondary to the question "What do we want to accomplish in terms of health outcomes?". Linking budgetary spending to outcome targets is not new. Since 2005, India has been using an outcome-linked budgeting process. But any such process is only as good as the data on which it is based and the analysis and work that goes into defining appropriate outcome measures.

With public health, it is possible to devise measures that directly link an action to a healthcare outcome. For example, vaccination has a direct effect on reducing the burden of disease. Ensuring that more mothers deliver their babies in an institutional environment has a direct favorable effect on reducing both maternal and neonatal mortality. Indeed, as measured in past outcome budgets, India has done well on these measures. But communicable diseases are on the decline (e.g., diarrheal disease in terms of "years of lives lost (YLL)" has declined 56% between 1990 and 2010) whereas there is a massive rise in YLLs because of non-communicable diseases. For example, there has been a 66% increase in YLL because of ischemic heart disease over the same period, a figure that continues to rise.

Unlike communicable diseases which are episodic, non-communicable diseases like diabetes and hypertension are lifelong afflictions that gradually increase in severity while also having secondary consequences that are disabling and expensive (both to treat and in terms of loss of earnings). The rapid growth in NCDs in India has the potential to cripple the economy. The solutions are not simple. The wicked nature of the causative chain of events that lead to NCDs means that measures to combat NCDs have to be complex and dynamic. The budget should have allocated a sizable chunk of spending to addressing this emerging epidemic. But the numbers belie this expectation. In 2021-22, the central budget allocated only INR 700 cr for NCDs against a more handsome 2900 cr for HIV-AIDS and STD control. Even more important is the failure to define target healthcare outcomes for the spending on NCDs.

So, how do we come up with Outcome Measures? The 2021-22 MoHFW Outcome Budget lists several salient measures for HIV. For example, the percentage of people living with HIV who know they have HIV (the targeted outcome is 90%). Having such discrete and targetable outcome measures has been behind India's success in combating communicable diseases. We need to think about doing the same for NCDs. For NCDs, devising outcome measures that can be tracked at scale is difficult given the polymorphic nature of these conditions (e.g., complications of NCDs can affect almost every organ in the body) and their complex interaction with environmental and lifestyle factors. But, using hypertension as an example, we could have outcome measures like the percentage of hypertensives who know they have hypertension, the percentage of hypertensives who are receiving treatment, the percentage of treated hypertensives who are within the ideal range for blood pressure, etc. Revealingly, under the National Program for Prevention and Control of Cancer, Diabetes, Cardiovascular Diseases and Stroke (NPCDCS), there are no clinical outcome targets set.

Making the healthcare budget salient to current needs is a self-evident priority. But this gets derailed by three problems inherent to the budgeting process. Firstly, there is a lack of coordination between central spending and state spending on healthcare. India's accomplishments in communicable diseases are due to strong centrally led and coordinated mission-mode programs. Such mission-mode approaches should be implemented for the big killers of non-communicable diseases as well. But before swamping such missions with loads of money, there should be careful forethought given to the health outcomes being targeted as well as the means to measure them longitudinally. Performance on these programs should be part of a National Health Survey that should be presented alongside the National Economic Survey. A critical input for such an outcome-driven budgeting process will be the availability of rich data on clinical status and outcomes at the community level.

If in other sectors data is gold, in healthcare data is diamond. Digitally enabled collection and analysis of healthcare data can inform our budgeting process and make it soundly evidence based. The potential savings for the Indian economy, both by eliminating wasteful (and harmful) expenditure and by improving efficiency could be in thousands of Crores. The National Digital Health Mission (NDHM) is a step in the right direction. But it has to be even more ambitious, given its potential to generate positive outcomes of such magnitude. The minuscule allocation of 200 Crs toward NDHM pales in comparison to the 1000 crore annual budget that was allocated for the implementation of Aadhaar, indicating that the Government has not taken seriously the potential for digital medicine to transform the landscape for healthcare in India. The resources committed to digital health have to be much greater because it has a higher level of complexity. Front loading this spend can accelerate the capture of the efficiency and economic gains that result from digitalization, freeing up more resources down the road. The availability of high-quality data from NDHM can be the keystone supporting a rational and demand-led budgeting process for healthcare in which allocations are coupled to outcomes. This is common sense. But in the corridors of Government and Politics, it takes many cries of the "emperor is naked" to get change going.

03 | WHY INDIA SHOULD NOT GO THE NHS WAY

"People are dying after waiting for hours; staff talk of ending it all': Inside the NHS crisis 'warzone' – headline from The Manchester Evening News, 22 January 2023

Since we wrote the the piece that follows, the unpreparedness of the NHS for what lies in its near future, is becoming clearer (The Economist 27 May 2023; To survive, Britain's NHS must stop fixating on hospital care). Doctors and nurses in the UK are up in arms against the NHS authority, and there is high attrition among doctors and nurses. Hospital waiting lists are growing (above 7 million) along with growth in inappropriate use of emergency care. One in 11 posts in the NHS lies vacant. Britain also has the worst 5-year survival rates for many cancers and poorer outcomes for heart attacks and strokes among 18 OECD members. The piece in The Economist calls for increased spending on healthcare, targeting primary care. In other words, the NHS often held up as a paragon for other countries to follow is having its problems. But we should not throw the baby out with the bathwater, there are many aspects of the NHS, such as comprehensive, universal, and free at the point of delivery care that are valued by British citizens. The NHS needs a dose of radical reform. The Economist proposes a greater emphasis on community care versus the current budget-driven emphasis on hospital care. The article mentions Community Care, Decentralization, and Technology (that unifies patient data) as possible solutions. These ideas resonate with some of the thoughts we have shared, but these alone will not do the trick. Much more than those three interventions are needed, and we have provided some options for additional interventions as well - such as focused factories and managed competition as ways to get the best of a hybrid system combining government and private delivery into one unified system of healthcare that is not driven by consumption but by clinical outcomes. The measures call for the kind of bold imagination that cannot appear on the pages of a mainstream publication.

In the piece titled "A national health service in India" (The Hindu, Comment: May 10, 2021), Prof. Arvind Sivaramakrishnan puts forth the view that India needs a health system modeled on the National Health Service of the UK. This is a popular view that is reinforced by calls made during the ongoing pandemic to nationalize healthcare in India. This is also the view put forward in the Bhore Committee report (1946), which served as a blueprint for the development of healthcare services in India post-independence. While we agree that the current laissez-faire capitalism in healthcare must go, our conclusions are at variance with Prof. Sivaramakrishnan's recommendation on what should replace the current system.

The NHS is a taxpayer-funded healthcare system that is free for every citizen of the United Kingdom. It is appealing in its simplicity: there is a single-payer—the government—and administrative costs at 16% of healthcare spending are much lower than the 25% it costs to administer healthcare in the US. The NHS is so loved by British citizens that it has been described as the "national religion". It is no wonder that the NHS is held up as an example of a well-run healthcare system worthy of emulation by other nations.

If we could rewind to when the Bhore committee made its recommendations, it is possible to visualize India slowly building up a system of healthcare resembling the NHS. But 73 years have passed, and we have strayed too far from our post-independence trajectory to make a convenient U-turn. Private healthcare dominates the landscape in India, accounting for over 75% of healthcare spending and 65% of hospital beds. We cannot wish away this legacy. Any system that replaces our current healthcare system must incorporate this legacy within its fold.

A nationalized healthcare system will pose a second challenge. Indian Government hospitals are not paragons of virtue. Although free, the people they are supposed to serve shun them. Even our leaders, politicians and bureaucrats, do not have faith in them. Except for a few elite institutions, much of Government healthcare, especially primary care, falls short of delivering acceptable levels of quality. In such a situation, expecting the Government to replicate the NHS here in India would be a pipe dream.

So, what could such an alternate system be that could replace what we have? First, we see a large role for the Government in any new system, especially in a system of Universal Health Coverage in which no citizen is denied healthcare because of inability to pay.

The primary role of the Government should be as an "enlightened" regulator of healthcare. Fortunately, we have good examples of how the Government has played the role of an enlightened regulator — the SEBI, which is described as a "watchful and efficient regulator" of the securities market, being a prime example. Like the SEBI, a healthcare regulator will also have to bring transparency into the workings of the healthcare marketplace. Since Clinical Outcomes and Costs are paramount, we will need our healthcare institutions to be completely transparent on these two measures. The national healthcare information technology backbone that has been announced can be a key enabler in bringing healthcare data from both private and public institutions out in the open for the regulator to analyze as a basis for setting standards and monitoring performance.

Apart from this, the Government should also operate the core of healthcare - comprising primary healthcare, as well as emergency care centers. Government primary healthcare (which we label Comprehensive Care in Section 1) will serve as a gatekeeper to access tertiary care and coordinate care received by an individual throughout her lifetime. Government-run facilities will also provide emergency care. On the other hand, private players will provide all elective care, where both costs and outcomes are predictable. This can be based on fixed-price contracts, not unlike the current Ayushman Bharat model.

Such a mixed model will do several things—it will effectively control costs and quality through the disciplining role of the Government-run components; it will make the best use of capacity in the private system, thus allowing an element of marketplace competition and improving efficiency while ensuring through negotiated price-fixing that costs do not run away as in the current opaque fee-for-service system. Thus, the arrangement provides for a "best of both worlds" scenario.

The principles of such a mixed system should be (1) move as much of healthcare as possible to value-based care (payment for clinical outcomes) from fee-for-service care (payment for a service that does not consider the value of the service in terms of the clinical outcome generated) (2) all predictable/elective care should be contracted to private players (3) there should be healthy transparency on metrics of performance, with a focus on clinical outcomes (4) fair competition from multiple players/business models should be encouraged with a level playing field.

In our view, this model comes closest to controlling costs while maintaining quality within a framework of Universal Health Coverage.

04 | IS UNIVERSAL HEALTHCARE DOABLE?

Everyone agrees that Universal Health Coverage (UHC) is a necessary good. But detail is lacking on how to get there. Vijay Chandru and Sharad Sharma, in a newspaper piece (Hindustan Times, August 11, 2021), have called for a "Moonshot" in healthcare and have projected a monthly expenditure of Rs. 1250 per Indian to achieve Universal Health Coverage by 2030 (or 22-lakh crore rupees for the projected 2030 population of 150 Crs). Let us examine the 22-lakh crore rupee figure a little closely. If we are to achieve anything like the UK-NHS standard of UHC where the current annual per capita spend is GBP 3227, then after correcting for purchasing power, the per capita figure for healthcare spend per annum would be closer to rupees one lakh today. At a country level, this would be 152 lakh Crs or 20% of India's GDP in 2030. We have to ask ourselves if the Indian economy can bear this cost. Is Rs. 1250 per month per Indian sufficient to deliver UHC, and if not, what is needed to support the much higher figure that we estimate? It is one thing to extrapolate a number from the present into the future, but a much more complex exercise to enumerate the actions that will make our UHC aspiration come true. We need a detailed road-map that will realistically take us toward UHC from where we are today. This road-map has to accommodate the realities of healthcare in India.

Any exercise that plots a course toward UHC should start by outlining a set of principles. The reason for this is simple: when we tinker with something as complex and rooted in legacy as healthcare, every change will bring about roll-on effects on other parts of the value chain that can negate the intended positive impact of the intervention. We need to think this through carefully and start with a set of simple principles that can guide our decisions and choices. We have been considering these issues, and what follows is our take on what some of these guiding principles might be. We should not consider these as either comprehensive or sacred, but simply as ideas that merit discussion of the kind required when dealing with something as complex as Universal Health Coverage.

Make volume an advantage: If there is one key and distinguishing characteristic of the Indian healthcare marketplace, it is volume. We have the largest concentrated volumes of patients in many diseases (including diseases thought of as afflicting the Western world, like diabetes and cancer). Our healthcare delivery system should respond by creating large, focused care facilities that can take advantage of economies of scale while leveraging volumes to improve the quality of care and clinical outcomes (higher-volume medical facilities produce better outcomes for patients). High-volume care also promotes efficient use of scarce resources such as specialists and costly medical equipment. Thus, superior clinical outcomes can be achieved at a lower unit cost. The Arvind Eyecare factory (an example of a focused factory) demonstrates how this works, and similarly, we have seen this in cardiac care (Narayana Health) and diabetes care (Dr. Mohan's Diabetes Specialties).

Government-provided Backbone: We cannot build UHC without the Government acting as the orchestrator. The Government has to play its role in establishing the rules for fair competition and set standards for quality while also operating gatekeeper functions (e.g. primary care) and emergency services.

Hybrid Business Models and New Business Models: India has a rich legacy of privately owned healthcare facilities that must be marshaled and incorporated into the UHC ecosystem, going beyond mere fund transfers for procedures done. Both for-profit and not-for-profit organizations must operate side by side and compete. Newer business models, e.g. physician-run cooperatives, must be seeded and encouraged, given that experience has shown in other countries that physician-owned and managed enterprises perform better than pure corporate models in healthcare delivery.

Transparency: Healthcare generates enormous amounts of data that can help understand trends, set pricing, monitor compliance, and assist consumers in shopping for the best care at the best price. While the individual patient's data will be owned by the patient and shared with explicit consent, both aggregate data, and data stripped of identifiers should be part of a vast and growing pool of data that can be used for research. Transparency will also go a long way toward reducing waste, fraud, and error in medical care.

Task shifting: We already have a severe shortage of specialists that is not going away anytime soon. Any roadmap toward UHC that is expected to increase the consumption of healthcare has to take this fact into account and institutionalize and facilitate the shifting of common medical tasks and even basic primary care to trained medical personnel who are not necessarily physicians. Liberating the time of highly trained physicians will allow them to perform higher-order tasks that are matched to their training, thus reducing the overall need for doctors.

Governance: The management of UHC will need the able administration of a cadre of medically trained administrators and business leaders. An Indian Medical Service, corresponding to the Indian Administrative Service, should be in place to train doctors to perform nonmedical roles with high efficiency.

One Standard of care for everyone, with rationing when required: UHC has to ensure that the same standard of care applies across the board regardless of the socioeconomic status of the patient. There will be limitations to this principle due to the finite nature of resources. But when expensive or difficult-to-get treatments are rationed, such rationing should not discriminate between individuals based on factors irrelevant to the medical context.

Payer Models: A monolithic NHS-like model will take decades to create and may not even be the best option. It would be better to allow those who can afford it to pay for their healthcare through insurance (private or public), thus reducing the expenditure burden on the Government.

These principles should not be written in stone. They should evolve and change as more data becomes available for analysis. However, having such principles as guideposts allows safe and ethical experimentation. The experiments we do should not simply be a test and fail model, but an iterative process that drives the evolution of ideas about what works best in healthcare.

Universal Health Coverage is doable, but *en route* to that goal, many complex issues will need solutions. Finding these solutions will require deep thinking, analysis, and experimentation. We have to stop thinking simply in terms of how much we will need to spend on healthcare. We need to think deeply about the important and hard-to-measure clinical outcomes that the expenditure is expected to deliver. A term like "Moonshot" helps achieve big and audacious short-term goals where resources are plentiful, such as the situation when the USA put a man on the moon. But the "Moonshot" mindset does not help in plotting a multi-decadal journey through the complex thicket of problems that healthcare poses. We need to keep this in mind as we begin the journey.

05 | IS PRIVATE EQUITY THE MEDICINE THAT INDIAN HEALTHCARE NEEDS?

Private equity (PE) funds acquire companies (usually under-performers), improve their performance, and then sell them at a higher price to new buyers (value unlocking). Profitability is improved by revenue management (e.g., focusing on higher-margin services), market consolidation (e.g., acquiring competitors), selling less productive assets (e.g., selling a facility in a low-income area), reducing operating costs (e.g., headcount), etc. Most of these strategies are short-term since the PE fund has only a few years to accomplish all this and exit its investment. As may be expected with such short-term measures, while the business may improve financially and value is created for the investors, this comes at a price. For example, up-selling in a healthcare business will inflate bills without improving clinical benefits to the patient. Mergers and acquisitions do the same thing by eliminating competition. They also reduce choice and access for patients. The positive influence of private equity, i.e., injection of growth capital and the consequent discipline of the marketplace, may improve business efficiency and profits, but this comes at a price that is paid by the consumer.

Private equity in Indian healthcare

Private equity in India's hospital sector dates back to 1996 when Schroder Capital Partners (the private equity arm of Schroders) invested in Indraprastha Medical Corporation Ltd (IMCL-Apollo Hospitals Delhi) and Indian Hospitals Corporation Ltd (initially the parent company of Apollo Hospitals). The handsome gains made by Schroder when they exited their investment during the IMCL IPO in 1997 made Indian private hospitals look attractive as targets for other private equity companies. At that time (from the mid-80s to the mid-90s), India's private hospitals depended mostly on debt funding (not easily accessible, even with interest rates in the region of 20% for secured lending). The entry of private equity was a significant development for the sector, and in the last 25 years or so, private equity has penetrated this sector extensively and is a key ingredient for the growth of India's hospital sector. Most hospital chains, whether listed or not, now have private equity investors as shareholders.

The recent announcement of the Temasek-Manipal Hospital deal, which valued the 30-year-old hospital network at around Rs. 40000 Crs (pegging its revenue multiple upwards of 8, at a time when most other listed hospital valuations reflect revenue multiples of between 2.5-5), shines the spotlight on the role of private equity in India's hospital sector. Private equity executives wax eloquent about their interest in taking control of the operations of the hospital networks, whether it is a tertiary care behemoth like Manipal with over 8000 beds, a relative upstart like Marengo Asia Hospitals with less than 1500 beds, or a single specialty mother and child network like Motherhood, with as few as 500 beds. How deep will private equity penetrate India's hospital sector? And while the influx of capital will benefit the owners of these hospitals, how will it play out for Indian healthcare consumers?

Many of the private hospital networks in India came into existence in the last 35 years. Dominating this space are top national and regional networks like Apollo, Max Healthcare, Fortis, and Narayana. All are privately owned, with eight of them being listed companies, and all of them have private equity funds as shareholders. Despite the buzz around these hospitals, cumulatively they account for only around 50,000 beds (or less than 5% of the 1.2 million beds in the private sector in India). However, the share of revenues of these networks is much higher, at ~20% of the total revenues of private sector hospitals.

Private equity-owned hospital networks have grown from a couple of thousand beds in 1996 (when private equity first entered the sector) to around 50,000 beds today—an average annual addition of less than 2,000 beds. The reported cost of setting up a hospital bed measuring up to the standards of a world-class tertiary care hospital was around Rs. 1.0 million/bed in the mid-90s and has grown to Rs. 5-10 million currently (an annual increase of around 7.5%). The total investment made by these hospitals on increasing bed capacity was around Rs. 2000 million in the mid-90s and perhaps around Rs. 15000 million today. To put this in perspective, capital expenditure incurred by the government on health in 2018-19 (the most recent period for which data is available) was around Rs. 560000 million. The capex incurred by the private equity-owned hospital networks is around 2.5% of that figure. In a country where private healthcare is dominant, it would appear that the current level of investments being made by these networks is negligible.

Another aspect to be taken note of is that most capacity addition in these networks is not being created ground up. It is mostly through acquisitions, as part of their attempts to "consolidate" capacity. So, while the bed capacity within these networks has grown by around ~2000 beds every year, perhaps it has helped catalyze the private sector to add beds (propelled by the hope of getting acquired at some point by these networks, hungry to show growth to their PE owners through such acquisitions). However, the target audience for these hospitals—the thin sliver of the Indian population consisting of the urban rich—means that for the population they wish to cater to, the bed capacity addition is excessive, leading to bed occupancy rates of less than 70%.

A sophisticated veneer masks the price gouging

The general perception is that private equity-owned hospitals are created to provide high-end tertiary and quaternary care. Media buzz is around their ability to provide cutting-edge treatments for complex medical conditions. But the ground reality is that a large proportion of their revenues comes from the provision of secondary care, which even smaller physician-owned hospitals are capable of providing at a much lower cost—for example, general surgery and childbirth. Private equity-owned networks are making significant investments in birthing and ambulatory surgery centers, to be able to compete more aggressively with physician-owned standalone hospitals. However, in this process, the cost of treatment goes up. Procedures like cesarean sections and hernia repair often cost twice as much in these network hospitals when compared to standalone physician-owned community hospitals. The increased rate of high margin services like cesarean sections in for-profit hospitals (60% in for-profit hospitals versus around 20% in government hospitals) is a surrogate indicator for where the interests of those who operate for-profit hospitals lie.

Failure to create value for patients

As far as outcomes are concerned, there is a shortage of data in the public domain to make any meaningful comparisons. Listing only requires these hospitals to make financial data available. Data on clinical outcomes or the cost of services provided is not shared publicly. Anecdotally, not-for-profit hospitals deliver much better outcomes at lower costs than for-profit hospitals. For example, Aravind Eye Hospitals versus its competitors in the private sector. This is not surprising, given that the private equity focus is on growth, profitability, and market capitalization and not as much on the clinical aspects of delivering quality care that improves outcomes. Senior leadership in for-profit hospitals are incentivized to focus on financial metrics at the cost of other metrics. In any case, and for the same reason, hospital information systems are not geared to capture hard data on clinical performance. Even investments that are intended to drive patient traffic are not based on marketing clinical performance to the community but by dangling the availability of "rock-star" doctors who are hired at huge costs.

Private equity in healthcare: corrosive effects seen in mature healthcare PE markets like the US

There have been many studies carried out in the developed world that compare clinical performance outcomes in private equity-owned hospitals against those in not-for-profit hospitals. Private equity-owned hospitals do not deliver better clinical outcomes. Indeed, the opposite may be true. Research published in the American Journal of Public Health in 2001[3] documented the poor nursing care provided in investor-owned hospitals compared to not-for-profits. A RAND Journal of Economics paper published in 2002[4] demonstrated that when hospital ownership changes from non-profit to for-profit, the mortality of patients increases while hospital profitability rises and staffing decreases. For-profit healthcare as epitomized by private equity ownership is not good for patients.

Private Equity is not a public good

Private equity, even when invested in a public good like healthcare, does not itself become a public good. The owners of private equity serve Mammon. This should be obvious to anyone. But the manner in which PE in healthcare is being embraced with open arms gives the impression that, somehow, it will improve the delivery of healthcare in the country. The opposite may be true. By consolidating capacity and up-selling services, PE has the potential to have a pernicious effect on the consumer experience of healthcare in the form of higher prices and aggressive selling of clinical services with marginal or no benefit.

Private investments through PE have to be regulated in a manner that it does not drive over-consumption. Unlike say a consumer product, over-consumption of healthcare is not benign. It can have roll-on effects that can result in adverse consequences. We have to bear this in mind when welcoming PE into healthcare in the country. While healthcare in the country does desperately need capital, perhaps that objective is better served by public investments in infrastructure through funds raised in the form of taxes.

06 | CAN INDIA AFFORD UNIVERSAL HEALTH COVERAGE (UHC)?

On 10 October 2019, the UN General Assembly adopted a resolution committing member nations to achieving Universal Health Coverage (UHC) by 2030. The Indian Government has signaled its intent to implement Universal Health Coverage in India over the next decade. India's National Health Policy (NHP 2017) includes this goal: "the attainment of the highest possible level of health and well-being for all at all ages, through a preventive and promotive health care orientation in all developmental policies, and universal access to good quality health care services without anyone having to face financial hardship as a consequence." The road-map toward achieving this goal is a work in progress. One of the concerns is that Universal Health Coverage is not affordable for Low and Middle-Income Countries like India. In our research, we have triangulated evidence from multiple sources to build a cost estimate for UHC. Based on this estimate, we conclude that UHC is an achievable objective for India, although it may require deep structural changes in the extant healthcare ecosystem. In this article, we discuss these issues.

Beyond the moral, ethical, and constitutional imperatives that drive the state to care for its citizens, there are also practical considerations: In the absence of UHC, families get pushed into poverty and become a greater burden on the state.

Furthermore, productivity is impaired, denting GDP growth. India is among the countries with high Out-of-Pocket Expenditures (OOPE; percentage of national health expenditure that is spent by individuals and families from their own resources) on healthcare, as seen in Table 1.

Table 1

	Countries ranked by UHC SCI (a higher number is better)			
	Country	UHC Service Coverage Index	% OOPE share of national healthcare expenditure	Households with OOPE >10% of annual income
1	Canada	89	14.8%	3.8%
2	UK	88	16.5%	2.2%
3	USA	83	10.9%	4.5%
4	China	82	35.5%	24.0%
5	Mexico	74	41.6%	1.6%
6	India	61	63.0%	17.3%
7	Bangladesh	51	78.5%	24.4%

Table 2

	UHC SCI and Life Expectancy at Birth (All data for 2019)					
S.No	Country	UHC Service Coverage Index	Life Expectancy at Birth	DALYs/1000	Health Expenditure per Capita	As% age of GDP
			(Years)	(Years)	($PPP)	
1	Canada	89	81.8	273.4	5476	10.8%
2	UK	88	80.9	293.2	4765	10.2%
3	USA	83	77.3	338.7	11027	16.8%
4	China	82	77.1	268.7	815	5.4%
5	Mexico	74	75.1	272.0	1058	5.4%
6	India	61	69.9	336.4	242	3.0%
7	Bangladesh	51	72.9	270.8	130	2.5%

In Table 1, select countries have been ranked by UHC service coverage index (UHC-SCI), a composite score obtained as the geometric mean of 14 tracer indicators of health service coverage. Broadly, for the countries in Table 1, there is an inverse relationship between the UHC service coverage index and OOPE on healthcare. India with a UHC-SCI of 61 and OOPE% of 63% is at the bottom, just above Bangladesh.

Apart from economic costs, what difference does UHC make to health outcomes? Table 2 shows UHC-SCI against life expectancy at birth. Again, there is a clear trend for countries with high UHC-SCI to also have better life expectancy. In general, countries with high UHC-SCI also have high per capita healthcare expenditures, as might be expected. The outlier is the US, which has a significantly higher per capita healthcare spend compared to Canada and the UK and yet performs worse on UHC-SCI and life expectancy. The method of implementation of UHC impacts the efficiency of healthcare delivery and resultant clinical outcomes.

UHC-SCI, broken down into its components, shows that over the years India has dramatically improved in the areas of infectious disease and reproductive (Table 3; see next page), but not so much in the areas of NCDs and Service Access (Table 3).

Table 3

UHC SCI trend for India 2000-2019			
UHC SCI	**2000**	**2010**	**2019**
Overall	31	48	61
Infectious Diseases	8	30	71
Reproductive Health	56	73	72
NCD	46	57	63
Service Access	44	41	44
Global Rank on UHC SCI	143	135	121
India (DALYs/1000)			
Overall	501.7	399.9	336.4
Infectious Diseases	169.8	103.4	58.1
Reproductive Health	74.5	52.5	33.1
NCD	183.4	184.3	194.9
Healthcare Expenditure			
Per Capita (INR)	986	2464	3708
% of GDP	4.7%	4.1%	3.0%
Govt Share as% of GDP	0.9%	1.2%	1.0%

Through focused mission-oriented programs, India has drastically reduced DALYs due to perinatal disease, but the trend of growing DALYs due to non-communicable diseases (NCDs), which are much more complex and expensive to manage, portends a grim future. If a wealthy country like the US struggles to bring NCDs under control (US DALYs are comparable to India due to the huge burden of NCDs), then unless India takes drastic measures, the future can be catastrophic.

In the journey toward UHC, the Government has initiated measures that include schemes like Ayushman Bharat, alongside state-specific schemes. These schemes attempt to universalize healthcare coverage by covering fixed treatment costs at empaneled hospitals, including private hospitals, for certain procedures. For treatments not eligible under these schemes, patients who cannot afford private care have to rely solely on hospitals run by the Government. The capacity of government-run hospitals falls far short of the load of patients they are burdened with. Furthermore, even in Ayushman Bharat, the expenses covered by the scheme are the barest minimum acceptable to private delivery institutions and do not compensate the patient for lost wages, travel to the hospital, accommodation for an accompanying attendant, etc. These are significant barriers to accessing care for someone below the poverty line. This explains the low uptake of such schemes. Offering a bouquet of incoherent schemes with plenty of gaps is not the solution or a desirable path toward UHC.

The existing model of healthcare, which is dominated by private fee-for-service players, is poorly suited to cost-effectively provide UHC. If there is one lesson to be learned from the experience of other nations implementing UHC, it is to strengthen government-operated or managed primary healthcare and make it available as close to citizens as possible. Primary healthcare should serve a gatekeeper function that ensures that patients are referred only when appropriate for specialist, secondary, or tertiary care. While all villages in India may not be close enough to a suitably equipped Primary Health Center (PHC), care at the doorstep should be possible through a health worker tethered to the nearest PHC using the tools of tele-health. Emergency care may also need to be redesigned to be as accessible as possible in the remotest regions of the country. Building such a comprehensive network will require significant upfront investments, as well as systems and procedures to integrate existing private players.

To estimate the cost of providing UHC for the Indian population, we need estimates of consumption and costs per unit of consumption. The National Sample Survey Organization (NSSO) data provides estimates of both. But both being retrospective data based on a pre-UHC situation can only be taken as baselines and not as targets to meet. To estimate consumption, we can look at consumption data for a country like Canada, which has one of the more successful models of UHC. However, this data on consumption has to be adjusted for differences due to Indian demographics and DALYs. Canada has an older demographic. But India has a higher DALY number, suggesting that despite a younger population, Indians in general have higher levels of morbidity. The only way to address these countervailing consumption drivers is to look at consumption data in a situation in India that may be closest to what UHC in practice may look like. .

TABLE 4

Estimating consumption, unit costs and total per capita costs of UHC (based on data for 2017-18)

	CONSUMPTION		COST/UNIT CONSUMED (INR)		COST/PER PERSON/PER YEAR (INR)		
	OPD visits per person per year	Hospitalizations per 100 persons per year	OPD Visit	Hospitalization	OPD Visits	Hospitalization	Total
Healthcare consumption India							
In Govt facilities	0.57	2.36	918	27353	523	646	1169
In Private Facilities	1.33	2.44	888	51130	1181	1248	2429
TOTAL	1.9	4.8			1704	1893	3597
Healthcare consumption in Indian Rlys							
In own facilities	3	5.9	918	27353	2754	1614	4368
In other hospitals		1.9		51130	0	971	971
TOTAL	3	7.8			2754	2585	5339
Healthcare consumption in Canada	6.7	8.3					
Assuming consumption like Canada and Costs like Indian Railways	6.7	8.3	918	27353	6151	2270	8421
Estimating consumption based on DALY data and actual consumption in Railway Hospitals							
In Govt facilities	3	7.2	1000	30000	3000	2160	
In private facilities	1	0.9	1000	50000	1000	450	
TOTAL	4	8			4000	2610	6600

The Indian Railways with its 1.3 million employees spread across the country, with access to healthcare close to their homes through a network of railway hospitals and clinics, comes close to being ideal in terms of healthcare provision in India. If we look at healthcare consumption among railway employees and their families, we can see that it is close to the current consumption rates in Canada for hospitalization, but still only 50% of Canadian consumption in terms of OPD visits.

Using information from these sources, we have estimated consumption under UHC in India (Table 4).

We have increased the target OPD visits to 4 per year (from 1.9 in the general population and 3 among Railway employees and families). This is to account for a projected increase in consumption (as seen in Canada for OPD visits) as part of a preventive approach to health under UHC. We have bumped up consumption of hospitalization only marginally since we have assumed that hospitalization among railway employees/ families is at near-ideal levels (a patient sick enough to be hospitalized is unlikely to defer or delay treatment when the employer is paying for care). Thus, the figure of 8 hospitalizations per 100 per year is slightly higher than rates currently prevalent in the railway employee population and slightly lower than what is seen in Canada.

Once we have triangulated estimates of consumption (Table 4), we need to look at costs per unit consumed for both OPD visits and hospitalizations. Here the Railways' data again has a normative value. We have estimated OPD costs of Rs. 1000 per visit and hospitalization costs of INR 50000 per admission. Based on annual consumption rates, the total annual cost of healthcare per Indian works out to INR 6600 (at 2018-2020 prices). At current population and GDP levels, this works out to an aggregate amount of INR 900000 Crs or 5.2% of GDP, which is 80% higher than current spending levels, or 3% of GDP. Targeting such costs may be unrealistic today. However, if we were to project a comprehensive UHC system to be implemented by 2035, the same level of spending would account for 2-3% of projected GDP (at 2018-2020 prices) and by 2050 only around 1% of GDP. While this estimate is only a rough approximation, even a doubling may not be a significant burden on costs. If consumption stays where we project it to be, UHC would be a highly affordable public good.

One item not accounted for in this estimate is the likelihood that the establishment of new methods of operation required for UHC can create significant front-loaded capital expenditures. Another is the concurrent spending on social determinants of health, such as public health and civic infrastructure, which could provide a multiplier effect to the direct spending on health. On the other hand, we have also not specifically accounted for savings that will result from avoiding wasteful expenditures (through a gatekeeper mechanism rendered through primary and community care clinics, and near-universal substitution of generics in the place of branded products).

The analysis presented here is a beginning. Given that UHC should be a compulsory public good, we have attempted to show that it is also an affordable public good. While our estimates may lack the precision that can only be arrived at by conducting a large-scale bottom-up exercise, it holds out hope that UHC is feasible. It should provide the impetus to take definitive actions toward making UHC a reality. The most difficult structural element to execute will be the establishment of a comprehensive network of primary/community health centers whose staff are charged with being the first point of call for patients for their healthcare needs. The second structural change will be the necessity in any UHC system to build a strong backbone of government-led delivery mechanisms (the gatekeeper mechanism and emergency care being core to this element) that can work with and get the best out of private players.

For a large country like India with wide income inequalities, UHC is an imperative and not a choice. By adopting new structures and institutions, the cost of UHC should be well within the means of the Indian economy. The gains in productivity resulting from a healthy population can outweigh the cost of implementing UHC. We estimate the cost of lost productivity due to DALYs at INR 765000 Crs in the year 2050 (at 2018-20 prices). We estimate that the productivity gain from improvements in health under UHC would account for almost 1% of GDP.

The necessity for deep structural changes in how healthcare is operated is unavoidable. It is a bullet the Government must bite if UHC in any form is to be realized. We have not in this piece covered initiatives in the area of public health that can contribute to significant improvements in the health of the population, e.g. control of air pollution or the plentiful availability of recreation areas for exercise. Any move toward UHC must take a comprehensively inclusive view of health.

In summary, UHC is a necessary public good that is affordable for a resurgent India with an expanding GDP. The right question to ask is - "Can India's aspiration to become a developed country on the back of a productive labor force afford NOT to have UHC?"

07 | ALTERNATE BUSINESS MODELS

Healthcare is an economic sector where the profit motive that underpins corporate actions can have a corrosive effect. Ultimately, it is the taxpayer who foots the bill. There are self-evident reasons for the conflict between the interests of the healthcare corporation and the healthcare consumer. In a use-driven billing system, there is a perverse incentive to increase consumption beyond what is essential. Such overconsumption is not merely financially ruinous, but the additional consumption of diagnostic and therapeutic services also has a deleterious effect on health, which is counter to the very purpose of healthcare. Asymmetry of information between the prescriber and the consumer and the payer further distorts the picture by allowing the prescriber to slant the consumption more in their interests than in the interests of the unknowing consumer. Finally, the lack of a tight correlation between what is consumed in the form of treatment and clinical outcomes leaves many gray zones where the interests of the consumer are subjugated to the financial interests of other players in the value chain.

There is no simple way to eliminate the adverse consequences of a freewheeling and laissez-faire marketplace that stimulates consumption up to the point where financial constraints do not allow it to grow any further. The only way to control this is to link provider incentives to "best possible" clinical outcomes. Again, "best possible" has to be within the framework of what the society as a whole can bear; money is not an infinite resource, and every economy has to tailor conditions and definitions of what level of healthcare to provide its citizens under UHC within budgetary constraints wherein multiple competing priorities have to be ranked and served to optimally satisfy most healthcare needs of most citizens most of the time.

The fact that resources are limited while the needs are almost infinite is all the more the reason why we must adopt a system of delivery that maximizes the clinical outcome potential of every rupee that is spent, as outlined in the section on WaFEr. Beyond that, simple market-force-yanked consumption-oriented business models are neither ethical nor sustainable in healthcare. This is where value-based healthcare has been proposed as a means to deliver healthcare that creates value for the end user and the system as a whole, placing it above the narrow commercial interests of private for-profit entities that participate in the value delivery chain. Doing this is not a simple task. The transition to value-based healthcare has been tough for traditional for-profit organizations and healthcare providers, given the increase in scope to include disease prevention and wellness care. A prevention orientation means engaging with the social context and changing patient behavior, issues that the current "medicalized" healthcare environment is not very good at. So, we need organizational structures where some form of patient-centric and value-based care is a natural and organic fit with the business model.

The not-for-profit model is not new in healthcare. Healthcare, since medieval times, has been delivered in hospitals and hospices, where care was free. The corporate model of healthcare is relatively recent, growing in a big way in the mid-20th century and taking root in India only in the 1980s. The non-corporate for-profit model was supplanted by large, listed companies that were answerable to shareholders and therefore accountable for the distributable financial surpluses they generated, even if that meant taking shortcuts and cutting corners on delivery.

In most marketplaces, private for-profit players bring efficiency and attention to quality. Will a marketplace dominated by non-profits retain these virtues? The VA healthcare system in the US is a not-for-profit system that serves veterans belonging to the armed forces. It outperforms private healthcare on several measures: lower risk-adjusted mortality rates, better patient safety statistics, widespread use of EHRs that support data analytics, comprehensive team-based primary care with integration of behavioral services, attention to social determinants of health, and caregiver involvement. The VA system demonstrates the superior outcomes that a not-for-profit healthcare system generates. It also offers a healthcare model that can be suitably customized and deployed in a country like India. A pure-play Government-operated non-profit model like the NHS (UK) may not be suitable. In India, a mixed model that hybridizes the best qualities of different models of ownership may work best. Enumerated below are some ownership models and their characteristics:

1. Physician-owned

The physician-owned health delivery system is probably the oldest for-profit model. The association of the physician with the delivery system means that there is an interest in ethically preserving the brand. Most nursing homes in India are owned by physicians, and many of them deliver high-quality care. The problem with this model is that it is evanescent. Once the owner-physician retires, there is a loss of continuity of vision. This is sometimes solved by having family members join the service or by selling the service to another physician. Again, there is no guarantee of continuity of vision. Despite these shortcomings, there is merit in physician-owned delivery models, since they perform better than other models of care[5]. However, with the increasing complexity of care and the need to have a network of delivery centers, there is a need for a group practice model where many physicians join together to run a network of centers. Sometimes this is done in the form of a physician cooperative.

2. Physician and community cooperatives

A physician cooperative can blend the benefits of being physician-owned with the strength in numbers that comes from multiple physicians pooling resources[6]. The cooperative can also have, as its members, representatives from the community that is served by the cooperative. They combine the expertise of physician owners with the protection of consumer interests by involved representatives from the community. We are not aware of the existence of any such blended physician-consumer health cooperatives in India. It will take some effort to bring together the two stakeholder groups and design the system so that it optimally serves both stakeholders. This will be like AMUL being composed of members who produce the milk and the end users who consume the milk. There are natural tensions that are set up in such a model, but if the physicians themselves are simultaneously members of the community (i.e. users), some of this tension can be released productively through an alignment of purpose. A meta-cooperative (a cooperative of the regional cooperatives) supported initially by the Government can help foster and develop the regional cooperatives by providing management expertise, creating and sharing best practices, and consolidating purchasing power to negotiate lower prices on everything from the EHR platform to consumables and support staff.

3. Government-owned and privately managed

The hospitality franchise model is one where a brand owned by a corporate entity finds a local entity to operate the venture consistent with brand rules. If the Government can be the owner of a physical asset, like a hospital, pays a management fee to a private player to operate the health system according to rules set by the Government, then this could work very well. This would be similar to the operation of much of the work in passport offices in India by TCS.

4. Hybrid

The opposite of the above can also work i.e. a private player builds infrastructure (like a hospital building or an MRI facility) and leases it to the Government. Staffing at senior levels is a mix of Government (administration, rule setting, and oversight functions) while mid-level staff and support staff can be entirely contractors from private players.

5. Private barnacles on public infrastructure

This is a model in which the sub-components of healthcare are contractually outsourced to private players, e.g. a government hospital can outsource diagnostic support to a private laboratory wherein the Government doctors maintain a gatekeeper function on tests ordered and oversight on the quality of the test reports along with negotiated volume-based pricing.

6. Government owned and operated

Different models may be appropriate for different parts of the ecosystem. The focused factory model can be run entirely as per models 3 and 4. Comprehensive primary care is preferably run as Model 2 or Model 5 with allowance for oversight by members of the local community (in the case of a cooperative, users can be included as members of the cooperative along with providers). Solution shop components of the ecosystem, the multi-specialty tertiary/quaternary hospital has to preferably be Government-owned and operated (like AIIMS). The same goes for emergency care centers and acute care facilities.

While the pandemic has certainly played a role in refocusing attention on healthcare, particularly hospital care, we do not believe that the experience during the pandemic should be a major driver in conversations about the kind of healthcare systems we need. Even if pandemics become commoner, they will remain less frequent than the bread-and-butter illnesses that plague our population. While we do present our views on how hospitals can be strengthened for mass hospitalization events, we are more focused on how an escalating response can be enabled by creating supportive on-demand capacity that is also mobile. In one way, though, the pandemic has helped. It has created a sense of dissatisfaction with the existing situation and triggered the kind of soul-searching analysis needed if we are to build a new system of healthcare by re-purposing pieces from the prevailing system.

08 | WHAT THE PANDEMIC HAS (NOT) TAUGHT US

A pandemic stretches health systems to the limit. Luckily, this COVID-19 pandemic has spared India the worst. We had fewer infections and deaths compared to many developed countries. But, there is no guarantee that the next pandemic will be kind. We have seen the carnage in Europe and the US; we cannot afford to have a similar situation arise in India. Our already inadequate health infrastructure will collapse under pressure. As preparation for a future pandemic, it would be wise to see what we can learn from the current one. The unpredictable behavior of pandemics limits our ability to anticipate every eventuality. We could, however, craft some generic measures that would help in any pandemic.

The COVID-19 outbreak was first detected in China in December 2019 when it was limited to the province of Hubei. There was an opportunity right then to contain the disease. The Chinese authorities missed the opportunity, and the world is paying the price. This highlights the importance of an effective response at the start of an outbreak. The response has to be firm, massive and globally coordinated. If China had worked closely with the WHO to stop all travel into and out of Hubei, the spread could have been contained. A massive response, early in an outbreak, when the seriousness is still not apparent, is a difficult decision. Health authorities fearing collateral economic damage delay action until it is too late. Political compulsions in an autocratic communist state like China were an additional factor that delayed the response.

Through global multilateral organizations, we need to create a mechanism; let us call it the International Pandemic Prevention Pact (PPP) to cushion the economic shocks of early drastic interventions. The political price of not complying with the PPP must be made so heavy that countries, in their self-interest, rush to cooperate with the international community when they detect a disease outbreak.

In normal times, such international cooperation would seem unrealistic. But we are just winding down from a pandemic that has caused incalculable loss of human lives and economic activity. This should be sufficient proof of the need for a strict multilateral alerting and response mechanism.

In India, a total lockdown was implemented fairly quickly. It was effective because a popular prime minister used the media to good effect. But it was brutal for millions of migrant workers. Overnight, daily wage-workers lost jobs and were compelled to trudge home to their villages. The Government's reaction to the unfolding tragedy was inadequate. Free emergency rations and essential supplies were delayed. A better-planned entry into the lockdown may have averted the tragedy.

The Government did a good job providing a steady diet of news and information during the pandemic. The Aarogya Setu app was a good initiative, although limited public use of the app blunted its effectiveness. India must count itself among the few major democracies that did not muster a panel of reputable scientists, virologists, immunologists, and epidemiologists to take audience questions at public briefings. Indian media continued to play to the ratings. It was especially disheartening how a religious group was singled out for adverse commentary. The Government failed to firmly and publicly repudiate the combustible rumors and fake news circulated to cause communal divisions.

Despite a weak public health infrastructure, we seem to have dodged the pandemic bullet. Next time may be different. It is important to strengthen India's pandemic response mechanisms and not leave the outcome of a future pandemic to chance. This can be looked at in three parts. The first is the quality of Governance during a pandemic.

Governance during a pandemic

The response to the pandemic across different states was patchy. In some states, contact tracing, testing, and quarantining were diligent.

In others, it was perfunctory. A pandemic transcends borders, and no state can ignore what is happening across its borders. Therefore, there is a need for strong top-down governance by the agencies of the Central Government. A key aspect of Governance is leadership. India needs a standing Pandemic Response Committee (PRC) that can be activated at short notice. It should have representation from the scientific, medical, and administrative cadres, as well as political representation from the States. Rules should be laid down by the Central PRC, but implementation can be left to the States.

One of the tasks for the PRC should be to create model response playbooks. The current pandemic is caused by a respiratory virus. The next one could be an antibiotic-resistant plague. All likely scenarios, including some outlier possibilities, should be studied by the PRC, and stock response playbooks created.

The PRC should define a communication plan that ensures frequent updates to the public. Media should be monitored, and rumors suppressed. An embedded media team within the PRC could help ensure that reportage directed at the public is accurate and up to date.

The 19th-century Epidemics Act needs to be rewritten as a coherent document that addresses all aspects of pandemics. The Act must define the responsibilities and rights of private hospitals and provide fair and equitable compensation for their role in the pandemic.

Surge Capacity

The second aspect is the need to ramp up healthcare services in response to a sudden surge in demand. It would be too expensive to maintain permanent overcapacity. Surge capacity needs to be rapidly created in response to a pandemic. To some extent, this is possible by shifting beds from routine elective care to the exigent needs of the pandemic. Mobile capacity (beds and medical equipment) can be kept on standby and airlifted to places where the demand for care during a pandemic overwhelms local resources. Modular prefab hospital bed units can be stored and shipped to places where there is a need. Beds are useless without appropriately trained medical staff. Therefore, it is necessary to cross-train doctors, nurses, and other paramedical staff in intensive care so that they can be redeployed during the pandemic from routine duties to caring for critically ill patients.

Enabling a rapid science and technology response

The third aspect of a response is to carefully curate and build the science and technology capabilities that can be repurposed toward studying the pandemic and crafting an evidence-based response, including diagnostic tests, drugs, and vaccines. The ability to collect and analyze clinical data from patients in real-time during the pandemic is key. If treatment is provided in designated centers, then this would be a trivial issue of electronically centralizing patient records. If the pathogen is novel, then this data will be key to quickly understand the behavior of the pathogen and using this knowledge to design diagnostic tests and treatments. The governance of product development and approval under these exigent conditions must be predetermined as part of the playbook for the pandemic so that exceptions can be made to allow emergency use of tests and treatments.

However important it may be to prevent and manage future pandemics, this should not distract us from the present and ongoing task of building a robust public health system. If there can be said to be a positive outcome to the pandemic, it is this: it has altered the national mood toward healthcare in general and public health in particular. This new mood among the citizens provides a window of opportunity for Governments to introduce non-populist healthcare measures that will find wide acceptance among a public traumatized by the pandemic. The pandemic has also unmasked the inadequacy of public health infrastructure and forced a radical rethink of all aspects of public health, so that the much-needed radical reforms of the kind we point out here can be realized.

Simply spending more money on piecemeal pandemic measures without thinking through the multiplicity of interrelated issues is a foolish luxury that India cannot afford. The redesign of healthcare must be in the context of the fact that millions do not have access to even basic healthcare. Public health that prevents disease, avoids wasteful expenditure, and improves the quality of care for every Indian is paramount. Attending to public health needs can go a long way toward mitigating the effects of any future pandemic.

09 | EVEN AFTER COVID-19, WE WILL HAVE TO RATION HEALTHCARE.

The COVID-19 pandemic has foregrounded an issue that plagues healthcare and yet is rarely discussed: rationing in the provision of healthcare. When COVID-19 death rates peaked in Italy in March 2020, TV channels flashed horrific images of desperate patients lined up in hospital corridors awaiting admission, even as overworked healthcare workers triaged the arriving rush. It isn't as if the doctors had a playbook to make decisions about who got a bed and who had to be sent home. They had to extemporize on their feet, knowing fully well that some of those sent home might die.

The arrival of COVID-19 in India in late March 2020 sparked fears of a cataclysmic crisis given the inadequacy of the health infrastructure, the largely poor living conditions, and the density of the population. In Maharashtra and Delhi, the worst-hit parts of the country, ventilators, ICU beds, nurses, doctors, and medicines were all in short supply at different points. Some patients died while shuttling from one hospital to another in search of a bed. But fortunately, many of our worst fears did not come to pass – perhaps more due to luck, since the fatality rate in India was lower than expected.

Now, with the launch of a vaccine, the next phase of COVID-19-related rationing will happen if there is a sudden surge in COVID cases due to a new variant. The vaccine is manufactured in batches, so an instantaneous roll-out to the entire population is impossible. The initial vaccination campaigns have to target those most at risk – the elderly and healthcare workers. Some who are eager to be vaccinated so that they can safely return to work will have to wait. If it is simply left to the market, vaccine supplies will be cornered by the rich and the powerful. There may even be a black market in vaccine supplies. To avoid these problems, we need to carefully plan and execute the rationing of initial supplies.

In 'normal' times, healthcare services should be sufficient to meet demand, and everyone should be served. The reality, however, is far from that ideal – not just in India but even in the OECD countries.

What is underappreciated is the fact that, especially in countries like India, even before the pandemic struck, healthcare was rationed because of the inability of public health resources to adequately meet demand. While this can be compensated to some extent by increasing spend and reducing wasteful expenditure, the truth is that even under the best circumstances, healthcare will have to be rationed. The impact of rationing can be mitigated if it is done in a planned, rule-based, and transparent manner so that the poor and voiceless are not deprived of their fair share of what the nation spends on the health of its citizens.

Rationing beyond COVID-19

The US spends the most among all countries on the healthcare of its citizens. Despite this, about six million Americans don't have health insurance. They find it difficult to get routine care and hence have to wait until their health has worsened sufficiently for them to be eligible to be treated in emergency wards. As a result, more than 26,000 Americans die each year, according to a 2008 estimate[7].

In countries like Canada and the UK, which have implemented socialized healthcare, routine outpatient care is available on demand, but elective procedures like joint replacements are accessible only after a waiting period that can last as long as six months. The enforced immobility due to a joint problem can, in the meantime, cause other health problems, and some patients may die waiting for surgery.

Rationing healthcare in countries like India is like an iceberg: much of it is invisible. The poor in India depend on free care provided by government hospitals. However, such care is extremely variable, both in quantity and quality. There are long waiting lists for surgical procedures. Costly medicines are not easily available, and doctors often have to choose who will get the medicine and who won't. Many poor patients are too illiterate to know that they are being provided substandard treatment due to a shortage of equipment and medicines. They don't have a choice, and they accept what they are given. This situation is so commonplace that it is too banal to be covered in the news.

A million Indians die each year because of an inability to access care[8]. If everything were equal and receiving costly treatment at a government hospital was simply a matter of standing in line, it may still be a fair system. However, extraneous considerations often influence who gets treated and who doesn't. How healthcare resources are apportioned also depends on gender, age, socioeconomic status, and caste. People close to power appropriate precious resources out of turn, precipitating even greater misery for those unfortunate who don't have a voice in the corridors of power.

If the shortage of healthcare supplies and services, and inequity in their distribution, is bad now, it's only likely to get worse. Specifically, three drivers will increase the pressure to ration healthcare in India's near future.

Growth in rationing of healthcare

For one, medical and technological breakthroughs are being produced at a breakneck pace. Many of the new treatments are far superior to existing ones – but such innovation comes at a price. Novel anti-cancer treatments can cost lakhs of rupees. An Apollo Hospital in Chennai has installed a proton-beam therapy machine, and treatment for one patient costs INR 20-30 lakh. It is impossible to imagine a scenario wherein the Indian public health system – even in an idealized future – can make such procedures available for free to all who may benefit from them.

The second driver is India's demographic transition. More Indians are living longer – but not necessarily in good health. Among the world's countries, Indians spend the longest period on average in sickness toward the end of life: 15 years. Much of this is likely to be expensive hospital-based care that strains our resources further.

The third driver that will compel rationing is the promise of the Government of India to move to a system of Universal Health Coverage. This should be accompanied by some increase in government spending on healthcare. The government itself has promised to double healthcare expenditure to 2.5% of GDP – but this won't suffice to cover a minimum acceptable standard for all those who depend on free care at present. In response, the government will have to even more tightly enforce rationing norms.

Equitable rationing

Rationing is inevitable, so can we make it equitable? First, if rationing is to be implemented, it has to be based on a set of rules rather than becoming the arbitrary choice of a front-line healthcare worker. Having sound rationing rules will also protect front-line workers from blame when rationing decisions come to favor one group over another.

A rules-based rationing system, in turn, has to be grounded in certain principles. The first is that the value of life can't be based on social and economic considerations. The life of a poor person is worth as much as the life of a rich person, and the life of a woman is worth as much as the life of a man. These principles bear repeating because, in practice, decision-makers often violate them. With such non-negotiable principles in place, we can then create a set of rules that account for local considerations.

A simple rationing technique that is consistent with this principle and is also easy to implement and resistant to corruption is a lottery system, whereby officials randomly pick those who can avail treatment. The problem with a lottery system is that it is blind to many other relevant considerations. For example, it won't distinguish between an 85-year-old in poor health who has only a few more years to live, and a 45-year-old with several dependents who is otherwise in good health. If both need an artificial joint replacement surgery, it is easy to see that when resources are limited, the 45-year-old should get preference. The lottery system won't take such considerations into account.

The same can be said of a first-come-first-served system, which will favor those who live near a healthcare facility or those who have the means to get there quickly – usually the rich. It can also be manipulated by those who have the power to influence the queuing system.

A common rationing rule is to prefer those who are sickest – as is already the case with organ transplants. While this rule will work well in a variety of situations, it may not be the best answer when a health-status assessment is based on the subjective impression of a doctor, and when the sickest patients also have the least chance of benefiting from the treatment (since their health is so compromised that a full recovery is unlikely).

Another common rule is to treat those who are younger and so have the longest life expectancy ahead of them. For example, treating a cancer patient who is 20 years old with a curative but expensive treatment might be preferable over treating someone with the same condition who is over 65.

Healthcare workers, hospital administrators, and government policymakers can consider many other rules. But the point is that the decision-making algorithms have to be thought through, and the government has to implement them transparently, and subject the system to periodic audits. Once a decision-making rule set is ready, a technological solution could help eliminate points of failure. For example, the government can implement a system that uses information extracted from electronic medical records to generate composite eligibility scores that will determine or guide who is to be prioritized. Then again, this is easier said than done, and has to be managed with considerable thought and even some supervised experimentation.

Consultation with Civil Society

The ethics and practical considerations that should govern how healthcare is to be rationed are complex and have to account for the local context of the community and the hospital where rationing decisions are being made. So it is important to involve members of civil society to participate in the rule-framing process so that officials can settle tricky ethical issues with their participation and inputs.

Implementing a rationing system that is a black box will not fly in a system where democratic self-governance is the norm, especially since the issues aren't purely of a medical nature. Any rationing system will create winners and losers – but the rationing decisions themselves will have to optimize outcomes for society as a whole. For example, if the system prevents those who may not benefit from treatment, then it would free up medical resources – beds, doctors, and nurses – for patients who have the highest chances of benefiting from the treatment. This would be a way to free up resources that would otherwise get locked up in Sisyphean medical efforts that keep a body suspended in limbo between life and death.

Importantly, a system to ration healthcare can't function independently of those who are responsible for implementing it. Doctors in government hospitals always struggle with rationing decisions, and some get it better than others. It is always tempting to buy the best equipment, although the same amount of money could save more lives when spent on scaling up a low-tech approach to treatment.

Dr. R. Venkataswami, a renowned plastic surgeon at the Government Stanley Hospital in Chennai from the 1970s to the 1990s, ran a world-class hand surgery unit that he built from scratch[9]. At a time when micro-surgical reattachment of amputated fingers and thumbs was becoming popular, he was confronted with a choice: to offer microsurgery as a first-line option or reserve it for those in desperate need, e.g. those who needed a reattachment of the thumb, a vital digit. While the temptation must have been great to focus on the former, Dr. Venkataswami knew that it would come at a steep cost: the inability to treat every patient, since microsurgery soaked up a disproportionate amount of departmental resources. A surgeon would spend upwards of six hours for each such surgery. Dr. Venkataswami made a conscious decision to limit microsurgery to cases where a critical hand function was at stake, and for the remaining patients, he resorted to more standard techniques that could be performed quickly and with fewer resources. By doing this, he didn't have to turn away a single patient coming to the department.

This kind of holistic planning and resource prioritization has to be standard training for all doctors, to prepare them for a world in which healthcare resources will be a zero-sum game. Putting it bluntly one patient's costly treatment will be another patient's inability to get treated.

Given the difficult ethical choices imposed on rationing decisions, the overall healthcare delivery system must be efficient and productive, so that we can minimize the need to ration. Our public health systems are a far cry from this. By reducing waste, fraud, and errors, we can take a big bite out of healthcare expenditure that can be reallocated to care that is necessary.

Big or small, the resources for healthcare are ultimately finite – but the demand for costly new treatments is growing rapidly. We must extract the most value out of our healthcare budgets so that the pain and deprivation imposed by rationing are mitigated to the extent possible. Having done this, we should then install a simple, transparent, and easily implemented rationing mechanism in which our poorest and most deprived citizens can have faith, secure in the knowledge that they will not be denied treatment because of their socioeconomic status.

SECTION SUMMARY AND CONCLUSIONS

Here are some facts worth remembering when thinking about UHC:

1. As per SDG 15 of the UN, all member countries must implement UHC by 2030.

2. The UHC service coverage index increased from 45 in 2000 to 67 in 2019 (for India, this is 61; for the UK, it is 88), with the fastest gains in the WHO African Region. However, 2 billion people are facing catastrophic or impoverishing health spending.

3. Not-for-profit healthcare is not only cheaper but also produces better clinical outcomes than for-profit healthcare.

4. Cell therapy costs tens of thousands of dollars. Cell therapy will also be the fastest-growing treatment approach used in curative healthcare in the future. Even OECD countries have not figured out how they will offer this treatment to their citizens.

5. Every year, 70 million Indians get pushed back into poverty due to out-of-pocket expenditures on healthcare.

6. The gap between supply and demand for healthcare in rural areas versus urban areas is stark. In rural areas, there is a shortage of both medical personnel and hospital beds. In urban areas, there is an oversupply of both. And yet, in both rural and urban areas, patients go untreated. In rural areas primarily because of throttled supply, and in urban areas because the supply is too expensive for the average Indian to afford.

We have shown that UHC is not only affordable but is also essential if India is to achieve its economic goals. Indeed, the two objectives are intertwined. However, to achieve UHC, the Government will need to intervene strongly to set up a core gatekeeping function and also tightly manage the ecosystem using an algorithmic (and therefore predictable) managed competition system to control the quality and costs of elective care and procedures.

The system can allow private for-profit players to coexist with government and not-for-profit providers. Managed competition rules framed by the Government can be used to control unbridled consumption driven by profiteering. Alternate business models, such as cooperatives that are run by physicians and local governments together, can be used to assure quality care while rewarding healthcare workers fairly for their work. The overall focus has to be to combine the efficiency and innovation of private enterprise with the need to provide affordable, high-quality healthcare. It is only a lack of imagination that can lead us to believe that this is impossible to achieve.

It is not the cost of UHC that is a problem for India. The enormous burden of illness that will crush the nation if UHC is not implemented is the problem staring at us if we do not quickly move toward UHC in a time-bound manner.

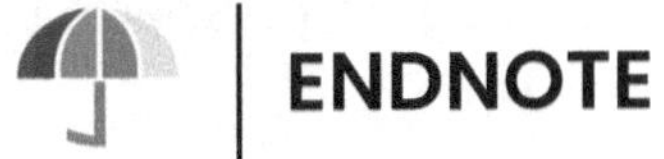 **ENDNOTE**

The strategy for moving to a high-value health care delivery system comprises six interdependent components: organizing around patients' medical conditions rather than physicians' medical specialties, measuring costs and outcomes for each patient, developing bundled prices for the full care cycle, integrating care across separate facilities, expanding geographic reach, and building an enabling IT platform.

M Porter and T Lee in "The Strategy that will fix healthcare", Harvard Business Review October 2013

"Only a crisis, actual or perceived, produces real change. When that crisis occurs, the actions that are taken depend on the ideas that are lying around. That, I believe, is our basic function: to develop alternatives to existing policies, to keep them alive and available until the politically impossible becomes the politically inevitable."

Milton Friedman, American economist and statistician

ENDNOTE: TEN BROAD RECOMMENDATIONS

Much of what we say in this book can be termed as common sense. Indeed, the quote from Porter and Lee at the start of this section summarizes pithily many of the points we make in this book. Where we have gone further is in proposing concrete measures relevant to India that give shape to the practical implementation of those principles.

The key implementation measures are as follows:

1. We need to re-imagine the role of primary healthcare. The new vision of primary healthcare that we paint is more appropriately called Comprehensive Care. Apart from performing the traditional

gatekeeper function, it will also have a 360-degree perspective, delivering, or coordinating, all healthcare needs.

2. We see a new and expanded role for Community Health Workers delivering care at the front-lines and in the homes. We also see them playing a role in providing resuscitative/stabilizing care for acute emergencies in places where traveling to the nearest emergency care center may not be possible within the golden hour.

3. The institutions that provide tertiary care must be dis-aggregated so that some will be focused care facilities that provide elective care focused on one class of medical conditions, like joint replacement or ischemic heart disease or organ transplantation. Such focused care facilities must treat a high volume of patients and use standardized protocols and extensive task shifting to control costs, while achieving high levels of efficiency and quality.

4. All kinds of waste, fraud, and error in healthcare must be controlled, or at least made negligible contributors to the cost of healthcare.

5. Health technologies (especially those that enable frugal care) and health information technology must be encouraged and deployed extensively so that information-based medicine becomes a reality. The Government must set standards and provide safe places (Health Innovation Parks) where innovations can be developed and tested in real-world conditions. Health IT must be used to force transparency so that patients are not disadvantaged in their selection of providers based on costs and quality. Remote care technologies and policies that allow front-line health workers to deliver some of the care currently in the sole purview of physicians must be strengthened as a national imperative.

6. A hybrid of non-profit and for-profit business models must be allowed to coexist with the following conditions: any solution-shop-style care provision (e.g. primary care and emergency care) must be run on a not-for-profit basis. Primary care (which we call

Comprehensive care in the form in which we envision it) must be fee-free to make it friction-less and support a preventive approach to healthcare. For-profit providers should be charged with delivering care for well-understood and structured problems, where care costs can be pre-negotiated in a rules based managed competition setting.

7.   The Government has a major role to play in all aspects of healthcare, ensuring progressive and fair governance that elicits the best clinical outcomes at the lowest possible cost. The Government's role must encompass setting standards and encouraging innovation in safe conditions that create a level playing field for innovators of all sizes. The vexatious issue of Central versus State Government authority must be resolved once and for all through a mechanism similar to the GST council, i.e., a shared process for setting policy, with policy implementation within pre-agreed boundaries at the State level.

8.   We need an institution like the UK National Institute for Clinical Excellence that can arbitrate on matters related to medicines and diagnostics and their reasonable use within a state-sponsored system of Universal Health Coverage. Such a center should be responsible for developing the evidence base for use and rationing of care decisions. Such an institute should also warehouse electronic healthcare data nationally for analysis, based on which recommendations can be issued.

9.   The point above leads us to a related point. Despite a confusing mélange of documents that the Government puts out in an attempt to paint a picture of Indian healthcare, the bundle of contradictions and circular references do not serve as a reliable compass for policymakers. Healthcare is like a supertanker. It cannot nimbly change direction. The trajectory we set today will influence the healthcare we get for years, if not decades. Hence, policymakers must have the right data. It should not be a difficult task for the Indian Government with its huge bureaucracy to take this up and

do a thorough job. While we await the day when all our healthcare data will be available in an easily accessible and analyzable digital format, we should, in the interim, put in place systems to measure and map what goes on in healthcare now. It may throw up some surprises that could influence the decisions we need to take on the journey toward UHC.

10. If we reviewed all the documents put out by the government over the years, starting with the Bhore Committee report, we will find that there are only a small handful of 'insights' in this book that have not been, in some fashion or another, explored in one or the other of the periodic reports. While there is a timidity in taking radical measures to fix problems, the bigger problem is the knowing-doing gap, i.e., a failure to translate insights into actions. There could be two reasons for this: (A) healthcare is a public good whose benefits play out over decades, thus making any incremental expenditures on new initiatives a casualty of pressing needs and political considerations, and (B) there is the lack of safe spaces for innovation and pilot initiatives to thrive.

For a complex area like healthcare, we must experiment with a variety of options before betting the house on one or the other. Such experimentation can inform the choices we make and thus help bridge the barrier between knowing and doing. Evidence from such experiments can also be the basis for building public and political consensus around choices that may cause pain in the near term but are vital if we are to achieve Universal Health Coverage. Our example of the Health Innovation Parks is a construct that is aligned with this kind of thinking.

The recommendations we make in this book may seem overwhelming, and they have to be if they are to bring about radical transformation. However, many of these initiatives can be rolled out in successive waves, allowing for the full digestion of the complexity of each initiative before moving on to the next one. Mandating e-prescriptions using existing infrastructure is feasible with small additional investments and can be accomplished in the next 3-5 years all over the country. As we describe in the chapter on PrescribeNET, the roll-on benefits for healthcare will be enormous, just from this one simple intervention. At the other end of the spectrum, building and deploying a Comprehensive Care network that becomes the default first point of contact for every citizen with a healthcare need will be a journey that may take longer. While building a nationwide Comprehensive Care network may seem mind-boggling in the first instance, we must keep in mind the following three points: (A) we do not have a better alternative if we are to make healthcare universal, (B) post-implementation, such a system will actually remove many of the existing complexities, such as patients crowding super-specialty hospitals for the simplest of ailments, (C) the long-term benefits we gain from a healthier population will far outweigh the short-term costs.

Finally, although we repeatedly make the point that the Government must lead the charge, we do not mean that the Government has to do everything. The Government's role is mainly to set standards and regulate. Beyond that, the "managed competition" model can be used to make the best use of private initiative and infrastructure. It would be a shame if we did not leverage the efficiencies and creativity of our private sector, especially the many healthcare start-ups, in serving the cause of Universal Health Coverage.

We cannot end better than by paraphrasing Arnold S. Relman from his book, "A Second Opinion" - If we have done our task properly, you will be interested enough in this book's message to want a wide public debate on the issues it raises. And if we have done our job really well, you may even be persuaded that the reforms we propose are necessary, feasible, and worth supporting.

REFERENCES AND READINGS

PREFACE

REFERENCES

1. Bhore, J. W. (1946). Report of the national health survey and development committee (Bhore Committee Report). Ministry of Health and Family Welfare, India, Vol. 1, 1–232. Retrieved from: https://www.nhp.gov.in/sites/default/files/pdf/Bhore_Committee_Report_VOL-1.pdf

2. Ministry of Health. (1961). MUDALIAR COMMITTEE: Report of the Health Survey and Planning Committee (August 1959- October1961). Government of India. Retrieved from: https://nihfw.ac.in/Doc/Reports/Mudalier%20%20Vol.pdf

3. Reimagining India's Health System: A Lancet Citizens Commission: https://citizenshealth.in

4. Arokiasamy, P. (2018). India's escalating burden of non-communicable diseases. The Lancet Global Health, 6(12), e1262–e1263. https://doi.org/10.1016/S2214-109X(18)30448-0

READINGS

Sarwal R, Prasad U, Madangopal K, Kalal S, Kaur D, Kumar A, Regy P, & Sharma J. (2021). Investment Opportunities in India's Healthcare Sector. https://www.niti.gov.in/sites/default/files/2021-03/InvestmentOpportunities_HealthcareSector_0.pdf

Section 1: THE ECOSYSTEM

REFERENCES

1. Churchman, C. West (December 1967). "Wicked Problems". Management Science. 14 (4): B-141–B-146. doi:10.1287/mnsc.14.4.B141

2. Kissick, W. (1994). "Medicine's Dilemmas". New Haven and New London, CT: Yale University Press.

3. The Sciences of the Artificial, by Herbert A Simon, ISBN: 9780262690232, Published: January 15, 1970, Publisher: The MIT Press

4. Christensen, Clayton M., Jerome H. Grossman M.D., and Jason Hwang M.D. The Innovator's Prescription: A Disruptive Solution for Health Care. McGraw-Hill, 2009.

5. Basu S, Berkowitz SA, Phillips RL, Bitton A, Landon BE, Phillips RS. Association of Primary Care Physician Supply With Population Mortality in the United States, 2005-2015. JAMA Intern Med. 2019 Apr 1;179(4):506-514. doi: 10.1001/jamainternmed.2018.7624. PMID: 30776056; PMCID: PMC6450307.

6. Starfield, B., Shi, L., & Macinko, J. (2005). Contribution of primary care to health systems and health. Milbank Quarterly. https://doi.org/10.1111/j.1468-0009.2005.00409.x

7. Levine DM, Landon BE, Linder JA. Quality and Experience of Outpatient Care in the United States for Adults With or Without Primary Care. JAMA Intern Med. 2019;179(3):363–372. doi:10.1001/jamainternmed.2018.6716

8. Phillips RL, McCauley LA, Koller CF. Implementing High-Quality Primary Care: A Report From the National Academies of Sciences, Engineering, and Medicine. JAMA. 2021;325(24):2437–2438. doi:10.1001/jama.2021.7430

9. The Hindu (April 1 2018) Union Minister of State for Health and Family Welfare Anupriya Patel, in a written reply to the Rajya Sabha recently, of the total 25,650 primary health centers (PHCs) in the country, 15,700 (61.2%) function with one doctor each. As many as 1,974 (7.69%) PHCs do not have even a single doctor.

10. Hayhoe, B., Cowling, T. E., Pillutla, V., Garg, P., Majeed, A., & Harris, M. (2018). Integrating a nationally scaled workforce of community health workers in primary care: a modeling study. Journal of the Royal Society of Medicine, 111(12), 453–461. https://doi.org/10.1177/0141076818803443

11. Grossman-Kahn R, Schoen J, Mallett JW, Brentani A, Kaselitz E, Heisler M. Challenges facing community health workers in Brazil's Family Health Strategy: A qualitative study. Int J Health Plann Manage. 2018 Apr;33(2):309-320. doi: 10.1002/hpm.2456. Epub 2017 Sep 21. PMID: 28940668; PMCID: PMC5934337.

12. Which Doctor For Primary Health Care? An Assessment Of Primary Health Care Providers In Chhattisgarh, India, June 2010, Report accessed at: https://cghealth.nic.in/cghealth17/Information/content/MediaPublication/WhichDoctorForPrimaryHealthCare.pdf

13. Healing Hands (paperback) by Swami Subramaniam – The inspiring story of the surgeon who set up the world's largest hand injury service and lessons for Indian healthcare (publisher: Swaminathan Subramaniam; available on Amazon)

READINGS

World Health Organization [WHO], & [UNICEF], T. U. N. C. F. (2018). A vision for Primary health care in the 21st Century. World Health Organization, 1–64. Retrieved from http://www.who.int/docs/default-source/primary-health/vision.pdf?sfvrsn=c3119034_2

Gupta, S., & Beckman, A. L. (2018). Strengthening primary care locally and globally: An interview with Asaf Bitton from Ariadne Labs. Healthcare, 6(4), 240–241. https://doi.org/10.1016/j.hjdsi.2018.06.005

Porter, M. E., Pabo, E. A., & Lee, T. H. (2013). Analysis & commentary redesigning primary care: A strategic vision to improve value by organizing around patients' needs. Health Affairs, 32(3), 516–525. https://doi.org/10.1377/hlthaff.2012.0961

Khemani, S. (2020). How India can lead the world to build a functioning public health system, (Figure 2), 1–2. Retrieved from https://www.ideasforindia.in/topics/human-development/how-india-can-lead-the-world-to-build-a-functioning-public-health-system.html

Orszag, P., & Rekhi, R. (2020). The Economic Case for Vertical Integration in Health Care. NEJM Catalyst, 1(3). https://doi.org/10.1056/cat.20.0119

Elrashidi, M. Y., Mohammed, K., Bora, P. R., Haydour, Q., Farah, W., DeJesus, R., … Ebbert, J. O. (2018). Co-located specialty care within primary care practice settings: A systematic review and meta-analysis. Healthcare, 6(1), 52–66. https://doi.org/10.1016/j.hjdsi.2017.09.001

Carroll A. The "Iron Triangle" of Health Care: Access, Cost, and Quality. JAMA Forum Archive. Published online October 3, 2012. doi:10.1001/jamahealthforum.2012.0058

Jeve, Y. B. (2018). Raising quality while reducing cost in health care: A retrospective cohort study. The International Journal of Health Planning and Management, 33(1), e228–e237. https://doi.org/10.1002/hpm.2454

White, W. D. (2002). The Changing Hospital Industry: Comparing Not-for-Profit and For-Profit Institutions. Journal of Health Politics, Policy and Law, 27(4), 692–696. https://doi.org/10.1215/03616878-27-4-692

Cook, D., Thompson, J. E., Habermann, E. B., Visscher, S. L., Dearani, J. A., Roger, V. L., & Borah, B. J. (2014). From "solution shop" model to "focused factory" in hospital surgery: Increasing care value and predictability. Health Affairs, 34(5), 746–755. https://doi.org/10.1377/hlthaff.2013.1266

Diwas SIngh, K. C. & Terwiesch, C. (2011). The Effects of Focus on Performance: Evidence from California Hospitals. Management Science, 57(11), 1897–1912. https://doi.org/10.1287/mnsc.1110.1401

Hyer, N. L., Wemmerlö V B, U., Morris, J. A., Wemmerlöv, U., Wemmerlö V B, U., & Morris, J. A. (2009). Performance analysis of a focused hospital unit: The case of an integrated trauma center. Article in Journal of Operations Management. https://doi.org/10.1016/j.jom.2008.08.003

Watson, D. E., & McGrail, K. M. (2009). More doctors or better care? Healthcare Quarterly (Toronto, Ont.), 12(4), 101–104. https://doi.org/10.12927/hcq.2013.21134\

Manes, E., Tchetchik, A., Tobol, Y., Durst, R., & Chodick, G. (2019). An empirical investigation of "physician congestion" in U.S. university hospitals. International Journal of Environmental Research and Public Health, 16(5). https://doi.org/10.3390/ijerph16050761

Measuring the availability of human resources for health and its relationship to Universal Health Coverage for 204 countries and territories from 1990 to 2019: A systematic analysis for the Global Burden of Disease Study 2019. The Lancet, 399(10341), 2129-2154. https://doi.org/10.1016/S0140-6736(22)00532-3

Carr-Hill, R., & Currie, E. (2013). What explains the distribution of doctors and nurses in different countries, and does it matter for health outcomes? Journal of Advanced Nursing, 69(11), 2525–2537. https://doi.org/10.1111/jan.12138

Auerbach, D. I., Chen, P. G., Friedberg, M. W., Reid, R., Lau, C., Buerhaus, P. I., & Mehrotra, A. (2013). Nurse-Managed Health Centers And Patient-Centreed Medical Homes Could Mitigate Expected Primary Care Physician Shortage. Health Affairs, 32(11), 1933–1941. https://doi.org/10.1377/hlthaff.2013.0596

Adams, E. K., & Markowitz, S. (2018). Improving Efficiency in the Health-Care System: Removing Anticompetitive Barriers for Advanced Practice Registered Nurses and Physician Assistants. The Hamilton Project, (June). Retrieved from https://www.brookings.edu/wp-content/uploads/2018/06/ES_THP_20180611_AdamsandMarkowitz.pdf

Lockwood, C. (2020). Nurses as substitutes for doctors in primary care. International Journal of Nursing Studies, 106. https://doi.org/10.1016/j.ijnurstu.2019.05.010

McMahon, L. F. (2007). The Hospitalist Movement — Time to Move On. New England Journal of Medicine, 357(25), 2627–2629. https://doi.org/10.1056/nejme078208

Hwang, J., & Christensen, C. M. (2008, October). Disruptive innovation in health care delivery: A framework for business-model innovation. Health Affairs. https://doi.org/10.1377/hlthaff.27.5.1329

Gupta, S., Palsule-Desai, O. D., Gnanasekaran, C., & Ravilla, T. (2018). Spillover Effects of Mission Activities on Revenues in Nonprofit Health Care: The Case of Aravind Eye Hospitals, India. Journal of Marketing Research, 55(6), 884–899. https://doi.org/10.1177/0022243718813347

Section 2: HEALTHCARE DOWN THE DRAIN

REFERENCES

1. Drug Price List: Generics and Matching Brands, accessed at: https://www.medindia.net/drug-price/index.asp

2. Lown Institute Hospitals Index: https://lownhospitalsindex.org/2021-winning-hospitals-avoiding-overuse/

3. Burnet, N. G., Mee, T., Gaito, S., Kirkby, N. F., Aitkenhead, A. H., Anandadas, C. N., Aznar, M. C., Barraclough, L. H., Borst, G., Charlwood, F. C., Clarke, M., Colaco, R. J., Crellin, A. M., Defourney, N. N., Hague, C. J., Harris, M., Henthorn, N. T., Hopkins, K. I., Hwang,

Fracr, E., … Whitfield, G. (2022). Estimating the percentage of patients who might benefit from proton beam therapy instead of X-ray radiotherapy. British Journal of Radiology, 95(1133). https://doi.org/10.1259/bjr.20211175

4. Sreevidya S, Sathiyasekaran B W. High cesarean rates in Madras (India): a population-based cross sectional study. BJOG. 2003 Feb;110(2):106-11. PMID: 12618152.

5. Gupta, M., & Saini, V. (2018). Cesarean section: Mortality and morbidity. In Journal of Clinical and Diagnostic Research (Vol. 12, Issue 9, pp. QE01–QE06). https://doi.org/10.7860/JCDR/2018/37034.11994

6. Kok, N., Ruiter, L., Hof, M., Ravelli, A., Mol, B., Pajkrt, E., & Kazemier, B. (2013). Risk of maternal and neonatal complications in subsequent pregnancy after planned cesarean section in a first birth, compared with emergency cesarean section: A nationwide comparative cohort study. BJOG: An International Journal of Obstetrics & Gynecology, 121(2), 216-223. https://doi.org/10.1111/1471-0528.12483

7. Chen, G., Chiang, W. L., Shu, B. C., Guo, Y. L., Chiou, S. T., & Chiang, T. L. (2017). Associations of cesarean delivery and the occurrence of neurodevelopmental disorders, asthma or obesity in childhood based on Taiwan birth cohort study. BMJ Open, 7(9), 1–9. https://doi.org/10.1136/bmjopen-2017-017086

8. Chavarro, J. E., Martín-Calvo, N., Yuan, C., Arvizu, M., Rich-Edwards, J. W., Michels, K. B., & Sun, Q. (2020). Association of Birth by Cesarean Delivery With Obesity and Type 2 Diabetes Among Adult Women. JAMA Network Open, 3(4), e202605. https://doi.org/10.1001/jamanetworkopen.2020.2605

READINGS

Kruk, M. E., Gage, A. D., Joseph, N. T., Danaei, G., García-Saisó, S., & Salomon, J. A. (2018). Mortality due to low-quality health systems in the Universal

Health Coverage era: a systematic analysis of amenable deaths in 137 countries. The Lancet, 392(10160), 2203–2212. https://doi.org/10.1016/S0140-6736(18)31668-4

Chalmers, K., Smith, P., Garber, J., Gopinath, V., Brownlee, S., Schwartz, A. L., … Saini, V. (2021). Assessment of Overuse of Medical Tests and Treatments at US Hospitals Using Medicare Claims. JAMA Network Open, 4(4), 1–13. https://doi.org/10.1001/jamanetworkopen.2021.8075

DuBois, J. M., Chibnall, J. T., Anderson, E. E., Walsh, H. A., Eggers, M., Baldwin, K., & Dineen, K. K. (2017). Exploring unnecessary invasive procedures in the United States: A retrospective mixed-methods analysis of cases from 2008-2016. Patient Safety in Surgery, 11(1), 1–12. https://doi.org/10.1186/s13037-017-0144-y

Yang, L., Liu, C., Wang, L., Yin, X., & Zhang, X. (2014). Public reporting improves antibiotic prescribing for upper respiratory tract infections in primary care: A matched-pair cluster-randomized trial in China. Health Research Policy and Systems, 12(1). https://doi.org/10.1186/1478-4505-12-61

Goel, R. K. (2021). Are health care scams infectious? Empirical evidence on contagion in health care fraud. Managerial and Decision Economics, 42(1), 198–208. https://doi.org/10.1002/mde.3224

Atul Gawande. (2015). America's Epidemic of Unnecessary Care | The New Yorker. Retrieved May 14, 2021, from https://www.newyorker.com/magazine/2015/05/11/overkill-atul-gawande?utm_source=NYR_REG_GATE

Lallemand, N. C. (2012). Health policy brief: Reducing waste in health care. Health Affairs, 1–5.

Xavier, T., Vasan, A., & S, V. (2017). Instilling fear makes good business sense: unwarranted hysterectomies in Karnataka. Indian Journal of Medical Ethics, 2(1), 49–55. https://doi.org/10.20529/ijme.2017.010

Shrank, W. H., Rogstad, T. L., & Parekh, N. (2019). Waste in the US Health Care System: Estimated Costs and Potential for Savings. JAMA - Journal of the American Medical Association, 322(15), 1501–1509. https://doi.org/10.1001/jama.2019.13978

Berger, D. (2014). Corruption ruins the doctor-patient relationship in India. BMJ (Online), 348(May), 1–2. https://doi.org/10.1136/bmj.g3169

Panagioti, M., Khan, K., Keers, R. N., Abuzour, A., Phipps, D., Kontopantelis, E., Bower, P., Campbell, S., Haneef, R., Avery, A. J., & Ashcroft, D. M. (2019). Prevalence, severity, and nature of preventable patient harm across medical care settings: Systematic review and meta-analysis. The BMJ, 366. https://doi.org/10.1136/bmj.l418

Jha, A. K., Larizgoitia, I., Audera-Lopez, C., Prasopa-Plaizier, N., Waters, H., & Bates, D. W. (2013). The global burden of unsafe medical care: Analytic modeling of observational studies. BMJ Quality and Safety, 22(10), 809–815. https://doi.org/10.1136/bmjqs-2012-001748

Section 3: HEALTH TECHNOLOGY

REFERENCES

1. Herzlinger, R. E. (1982). Why Innovation in Health Care Is So Hard. Proceedings of the American Society of Clinical Oncology, Vol. 1(May), 139–140.

2. Roberts, J. P., Fisher, T. R., Trowbridge, M. J., & Bent, C. (2016). A design thinking framework for healthcare management and innovation. Healthcare, 4(1), 11–14. https://doi.org/10.1016/j.hjdsi.2015.12.002

READINGS

Berwick, D. M. (2003). Disseminating Innovations in Health Care. JAMA, 289(15), 1969–1975. https://doi.org/10.1001/jama.289.15.1969

Jain, S. H. (2017). The health care innovation bubble. Healthcare, 5(4), 231–232. https://doi.org/10.1016/j.hjdsi.2017.08.002

Meskó, B., Drobni, Z., Bényei, É., Gergely, B., & Győrffy, Z. (2017). Digital health is a cultural transformation of traditional healthcare. MHealth, 3, 38–38. https://doi.org/10.21037/mhealth.2017.08.07

Kelly, C. J., & Young, A. J. (2017). Promoting innovation in healthcare. Future Hospital Journal, 4(2), 121–125. https://doi.org/10.7861/futurehosp.4-2-121

Snowdon, A. (2020). Digital health: A Framework for Healthcare Transformation. https://www.himss.org/resources/digital-health-framework-healthcare-transformation-white-paper

NDHM Sandbox Enabling Framework. (2020). Retrieved from https://ndhm.gov.in

Herzlinger, R. E. (1982). Why Innovation in Health Care Is So Hard. Proceedings of the American Society of Clinical Oncology, Vol. 1(May), 139–140.

Section 4: MISSION POSSIBLE

REFERENCES

1. Bloom, D. E., & Canning, D. (1999). The Health and Wealth of Nations World Development, 1207-1209. (May), 287.

2. Enthoven A.C. The history and principles of managed competition. Health Aff (Millwood). 1993;12 Suppl:24-48. doi: 10.1377/hlthaff.12.suppl_1.24. PMID: 8477935.

3. Harrington, C., Woolhandler, S., Mullan, J., Carrillo, H., & Himmelstein, D. U. (2001). Does investor ownership of nursing homes compromise the quality of care? *American Journal of Public Health*, 91(9), 1452–1455. https://doi.org/10.2105/AJPH.91.9.1452

4. Picone, G., Chou, S.-Y., & Sloan, F. (2002). *Are for-profit hospital conversions harmful to patients and to Medicare? ABI/INFORM Global pg. 507. The Rand Journal of Economics* (Vol. 33).

5. Ted Cho, Andrew Meshnick, Jesse M. Ehrenfeld, and Brian J. Miller, "Cost and Quality of Care in Physician-Owned Hospitals: A Systematic Review," Special Study, Mercatus Center at George Mason University, Arlington, Virginia, September 2021

6. Goldstein, M. T., Kern Augustine Conroy, J., & New York, P. (2013). Physician Medical Cooperatives Using the Agriculture Model-Legal and Structural Analysis. *The Health Lawyer, 25*(6), 32–42.

7. Tanne J. H. More than 26,000 Americans die each year because of lack of health insurance. BMJ. 2008 Apr 19;336(7649):855. doi: 10.1136/bmj.39549.693981.DB. PMID: 18420687; PMCID: PMC2323087.

8. Kruk, M. E., Gage, A. D., Joseph, N. T., Danaei, G., García-Saisó, S., & Salomon, J. A. (2018). Mortality due to low-quality health systems in the universal health coverage era: a systematic analysis of amenable deaths in 137 countries. The Lancet, 392(10160), 2203–2212. https://doi.org/10.1016/S0140-6736(18)31668-4

9. Healing Hands (paperback) by Swami Subramaniam – The inspiring story of the surgeon who set up the world's largest hand injury service and lessons for Indian healthcare (publisher: Swaminthan Subramaniam; available on Amazon)

READINGS

Garg, P. P., Frick, K. D., Diener-West, M., & Powe, N. R. (1999). Effect of the Ownership of Dialysis Facilities on Patients' Survival and Referral for Transplantation. New England Journal of Medicine, 341(22), 1653–1660. https://doi.org/10.1056/NEJM199911253412205

Gray, B. H., & McNerney, W. J. (1986). For-Profit Enterprise in Health Care. New England Journal of Medicine (Vol. 314). https://doi.org/10.1056/nejm198606053142335

Book: Priced out by Uwe Reinhardt, Princeton University Press, ISBN: 9780691192178 Published: May 14, 2019, Copyright:2019

Goldstein, M. T., Kern Augustine Conroy, J., & New York, P. (2013). Physician Medical Cooperatives Using the Agriculture Model-Legal and Structural Analysis. The Health Lawyer, 25(6), 32–42.

Chakravarthi, I., Roy, B., Mukhopadhyay, I., & Barria, S. (2017). Investing in health: Healthcare industry in India. Economic and Political Weekly, 52(45), 50–56.

Bhattacharyya, O., Khor, S., McGahan, A., Dunne, D., Daar, A. S., & Singer, P. A. (2010). Innovative health service delivery models in low and middle-income countries - what can we learn from the private sector? Health Research Policy and Systems, 8(Lmic), 1–11. https://doi.org/10.1186/1478-4505-8-24

Devereaux, P. J., Choi, P. T. L., Lacchetti, C., Weaver, B., Schünemann, H. J., Haines, T., … Guyatt, G. H. (2002). A systematic review and meta-analysis of studies comparing mortality rates of private for-profit and private not-for-profit hospitals. Cmaj, 166(11), 1399–1406.

Not-for-Profit Hospital Model in India. (2021). https://doi.org/10.31219/osf.io/ba5vu

Chakravarthi, I., Roy, B., Mukhopadhyay, I., & Barria, S. (2017). Investing in health: Healthcare industry in India. Economic and Political Weekly, 52(45), 50–56.

Shulkin, D. (2016). Beyond the VA Crisis - Becoming a high-performance network. New England Journal of Medicine, 374(11), 1001–1003. https://doi.org/10.1056/NEJMp1502629

Hussey, P., & Anderson, G. F. (2003). A comparison of single- and multi-payer health insurance systems and options for reform. Health Policy, 66(3), 215–228. https://doi.org/10.1016/S0168-8510(03)00050-2

Klein, R. (1993). Dimensions of rationing: Who should do what? In British Medical Journal (Vol. 307, Issue 6899, pp. 309–311). https://doi.org/10.1136/bmj.307.6899.309

Truog, R. D., Brock, D. W., Cook, D. J., Danis, M., Luce, J. M., Rubenfeld, G. D., & Levy, M. M. (2006). Rationing in the intensive care unit*. Critical Care Medicine, 34(4), 958–963. https://doi.org/10.1097/01.CCM.0000206116.10417.D9

Leslie P Scheunemann MD, M. P. H., & MD, D. B. W. (2011). The Ethics and Reality of Rationing in Medicine. Chest. https://www.ncbi.nlm.nih.gov/pmc/articles/PMC3415127/pdf/110622.pdf

Verrecchia, R., Thompson, R., & Yates, R. (2019). Universal Health Coverage and public health: a truly sustainable approach. In The Lancet Public Health (Vol. 4, Issue 1, pp. e10–e11). https://doi.org/10.1016/S2468-2667(18)30264-0

Kenny, N., & Joffres, C. (2008). An ethical analysis of international health priority-setting. Health Care Analysis, 16(2), 145–160. https://doi.org/10.1007/s10728-007-0065-5

Verrecchia, R., Thompson, R., & Yates, R. (2019). Universal Health Coverage and public health: a truly sustainable approach. In The Lancet Public Health (Vol. 4, Issue 1, pp. e10–e11). https://doi.org/10.1016/S2468-2667(18)30264-0

Kluge, H., Hunter, D. J., Bengoa, R., & Jakubowski, E. (2018). Leapfrogging The Elephants: Making Health System Transformation Happen Faster, Eurohealth — Vol.24 | No.1 | 2018

Varkey, P., Horne, A., & Bennet, K. E. (2008). Innovation in health care: A primer. American Journal of Medical Quality, 23(5), 382–388. https://doi.org/10.1177/1062860608317695

Healing Hands (Publisher: Swaminathan Subramaniam, available on Amazon.in), by Swami Subramaniam: The inspiring story of the surgeon who set up the world's largest hand injury service

ACKNOWLEDGMENTS

We would like to acknowledge the following persons for taking time and generously sharing their insights on a wide range of issues healthcare in India is faced with

Dr. Harish Pillai, Chief Executive Officer, Metro Pacific Health, Manila (formerly Chief Executive Officer, Aster India)

Dr. Arjun Rajagopalan, Former Medical Director and Trustee, Sundaram Medical Foundation

Mr. R. Basil, Founder Chairman, CauseBridge LLP (formerly MD and CEO, Manipal Hospitals, Executive President, Apollo Hospitals Group)

Dr. Girija Vaidyanathan, Chief Secretary (Retd.) Govt of Tamil Nadu

Mr. Sumit Nadgir, Managing Director, PAG (formerly Managing Director, True North Co)

Dr. K Ganapathy, Member Board of Directors and President, Apollo tele-health Networking Foundation and Apollo tele-health Services

Dr. Sakthivel Selvaraj, Director, Health Economics, Financing and Policy at Public Health Foundation of India (PHFI)

Mr. Vijay Santhanam, Retired business and marketing leader, author, inspirational speaker and visiting faculty at IIMs.

Dr A.V Gurava Reddy, Chief Joint Replacement Surgeon, Managing Director KIMS-Sunshine Hospitals

and Dr. K Aparajithan, a friend and Former Director, Atul Limited, for his suggestions on improving the flow and many corrections.

We thank our families for the support and encouragement provided during the writing process.

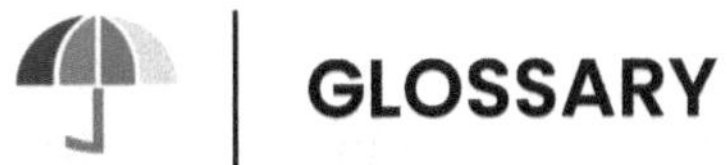 # GLOSSARY

Accountable care organization

An accountable care organization (ACO) is a healthcare organization that ties provider reimbursements to quality metrics and reductions in the cost of care. ACOs in the United States are formed from a group of coordinated health-care practitioners. They use alternative payment models, normally, capitation. The organization is accountable to patients and third-party payers for the quality, appropriateness and efficiency of the health care provided. According to the Centers for Medicare and Medicaid Services, an ACO is "an organization of health care practitioners that agrees to be accountable for the quality, cost, and overall care of Medicare beneficiaries who are enrolled in the traditional fee-for-service program who are assigned to it".

Ambulatory care

Ambulatory care or outpatient care is medical care provided on an outpatient basis, including diagnosis, observation, consultation, treatment, intervention, and rehabilitation services. This care can include advanced medical technology and procedures even when provided outside of hospitals

APR-DRG

All Patients Refined Diagnosis Related Groups (APR DRG) is a classification system that classifies patients according to their reason of admission, severity of illness and risk of mortality.

Average Length of Stay (ALOS)

The number of days (on average) that a patient spends in the hospital. To calculate ALOS, divide the total number of days in the hospital for all patients during a certain amount of time by the number of admissions or discharges.

Average Revenue Per Occupied Bed (ARPOB)

To calculate Average Revenues Per Occupied Bed (ARPOB), you need to divide the total revenue generated by a hospital over a specific period by the total number of beds occupied during the same period. Here's the formula: ARPOB = Total Revenue / Total Occupied Beds

Total Revenue: This is the total revenue generated by the hospital from all sources during the specified period. It includes revenue from services provided to patients, such as medical treatments, surgeries, diagnostic tests, room charges, and any other healthcare-related income.

Total Occupied Beds: This refers to the total number of beds that were occupied by patients during the same period. An "occupied bed" is one that has a patient admitted to it.

For example, if a hospital generated a total revenue of Rs. 10,000,000 during a month and had 500 beds occupied by patients in the same month, then the ARPOB for that month would be:

ARPOB = Rs. 10,000,000 / 500 beds = Rs. 20,000 per occupied bed

So, in this example, the hospital's Average Revenues Per Occupied Bed (ARPOB) for that month would be Rs. 20,000. This metric provides insight into how much revenue the hospital is generating for each bed that is being utilized by a patient.

Ayushman Bharat

Ayushman Bharat (AB) is an attempt to move from a selective approach to health care to deliver a comprehensive range of services spanning preventive, promotive, curative, rehabilitative and palliative care. It has two components which are complementary to each other. Under its first component, 1,50,000 Health & Wellness Centers (HWCs) will be created to deliver Comprehensive Primary Health Care, that is universal and free to users, with a focus on wellness and the delivery of an expanded range of services closer to the community. The second component is the Pradhan Mantri Jan Arogya Yojana (PM-JAY) which provides health insurance cover of Rs. 5 lakhs per year to over 10 crore poor and vulnerable families seeking secondary and tertiary care.

Care coordination

The organization of a patient's care across multiple health care providers.

Care guideline

Care guidelines guide healthcare workers through a clinical process or a task, e.g. the right way to measure BP or the drug with which to initiate antihypertensive treatment. They give general recommendations of how to perform a task, or advice on how to proceed in a situation.

Clinical outcome

Clinical outcomes are measurable changes in health, function or quality of life that result from medical interventions.

Combined Ratio

Combined ratio is a critical financial metric routinely used by insurance companies to evaluate their overall underwriting performance and profitability. The combined ratio takes into account both underwriting results (policy-related income and expenses) and investment income. It is expressed as a percentage.

The formula for calculating the combined ratio is as follows:

Combined Ratio = (Losses + Expenses + Dividends) / Earned Premiums

Comprehensivist

A term we have coined in this book to replace Primary Care Physician, since we propose that the Primary Care Physician role should be replaced by someone who can provide Comprehensive Care across many dimensions – speciality wise and temporal

Co-payment

A co-payment, or co-pay, is a pre-defined amount which the policyholder has to pay each time he or she gets a particular type of health care service. It is that portion of the claim which the insured agrees to bear in the event of a claim. The balance is to be paid by the insurance company.

Crore

Indian term for ten million

DALY

One DALY represents the loss of the equivalent of one year of full health. DALYs for a disease or health condition are the sum of the years of life lost to due to premature mortality (YLLs) and the years lived with a disability (YLDs) due to prevalent cases of the disease or health condition in a population.

Deductible

A deductible is an amount of money that the policyholder is responsible for paying toward an insured loss. Generally speaking, the larger the deductible, the less you pay in premiums for an insurance policy. A deductible can be either a specific dollar amount or a percentage of the total amount of insurance on a policy.

EHR

An Electronic Health Record (EHR) is an electronic version of a patient's medical history, that is maintained by the provider over time and may include all the key administrative clinical data relevant to that person's care under a particular provider, including demographics, progress notes, problems, medications, vital signs, past medical history, immunizations, laboratory data and radiology reports. Unlike an EMR, the EHR focuses on the entire health journey and contains a comprehensive view of the patient's health. In this book we use the term EHR since we believe any record should be comprehensive and not just a represent a slice of care as an EMR does.

EMR

Electronic medical records (EMRs) are a digital version of the paper charts in the clinician's office. An EMR contains the medical and treatment history of the patients in one practice. EMRs tend to cover specific illness episodes

EPO

Exclusive provider organization: a plan similar to an HMO that usually provides no coverage for any services delivered by out-of-network providers or facilities except in emergency or urgent care situations;

however, it generally does not require members to use a primary care physician for in-network referrals.

Focused care

A healthcare provider who provides only a single service, e.g. joint replacement or hernia repairs, is said to provide focused care.

Focused Factory

A factory that focuses on a narrow product mix for a particular market niche. Such factories will outperform the conventional plant, which attempts a broader mission.

Generics

A generic drug is a medication created to be the same as an already marketed brand-name drug in dosage form, safety, strength, route of administration, quality, performance characteristics, and intended use. Similarly, it is possible to have non-branded generic devices as well, although it is less common.

Health Information Exchange (HIE)

Electronic health information exchange (HIE) allows doctors, nurses, pharmacists, other health care providers and patients to appropriately access and securely share a patient's vital medical information electronically improving the speed, quality, safety and cost of patient care.

Health Savings Account (HSA)

A mechanism for taxpayers to deposit money in advance into a tax-advantaged account to draw upon for future medical expenses. This is used in the US.

HIPAA

The Health Insurance Portability and Accountability Act of 1996 (HIPAA) is a federal law that requires the creation of national standards to protect sensitive patient health information from being disclosed without the patient's consent or knowledge.

HMO

A type of health insurance plan that usually limits coverage to care from doctors who work for or contract with the HMO. It generally won't cover out-of-network care except in an emergency. An HMO may require you to live or work in its service area to be eligible for coverage.

Hospice

Hospice care is for people who are nearing the end of life. The services are provided by a team of health care professionals who maximize comfort for a person who is terminally ill by reducing pain and addressing physical, psychological, social and spiritual needs. To help families, hospice care also provides counseling, respite care and practical support. "Hospice" is a term from medieval times which referred to a place where travelers could rest (from the same linguistic root as "hospitality"), a way station of sorts where a person might be cared for by their hosts.

Hospitalist

A hospitalist is a doctor who provides care for patients at a hospital. They have the same education and training as your primary care doctor, but specialize in providing hospital care. They may also have other specialties such as pediatric (child-centered) medicine, internal medicine, or family medicine. A hospitalist doctor focuses on patient care inside a hospital, rather than on a specific organ or medical issue, like an allergist or a cardiologist does.

ICD-11

International Classification of Diseases 11th Revision · The global standard for diagnostic health information

Interoperability

IT systems that talk to each other so that data from one system can be ported to another easily

Jan Swasthya Abhiyan

The Jan Swasthya Abhiyan (JSA) was formed in 2001, with the coming together of 18 national networks that had organized activities across the country in 2000, in the lead up to the First Global Peoples Health Assembly, in Dhaka, in December 2000. The JSA forms the Indian regional circle of the global People's Health Movement (PHM). At present it is the major national platform that co-ordinates activities and actions on health and health care across the country. The JSA, today, is constituted of 21 national networks and organizations and state level JSA platforms (which are present in almost all states in the country). Network partners of the JSA include a range of organizations, including NGOs working in the area of health, feminist organizations, people's science organizations, service delivery networks and trade unions.

Keyhole surgery

Keyhole surgery is a technique that allows the surgeon to perform a procedure inside the body through a small incision in the skin. Some people refer to keyhole surgery as laparoscopic surgery, as it involves the use of an imaging instrument called a laparoscope to show what is inside the body.

Lakh

Indian term for one hundred thousand

Loss Ratio

Loss ratio is a key financial metric routinely used by health insurance companies that measures the relationship between the claims paid out by the insurance company and the premiums collected from policyholders over a specific period. It is used to assess the insurer's underwriting performance and profitability. The loss ratio is typically expressed as a percentage.

The formula for calculating the loss ratio is as follows:

Loss Ratio = (Total Claims Paid / Total Premiums Earned) x 100

Managed care

The term managed care or managed healthcare is used in the United States to describe a group of activities intended to reduce the cost of providing health care and providing American health insurance while improving the quality of that care ("managed care techniques"). It has become the predominant system of delivering and receiving American health care since its implementation in the early 1980s, and has been largely unaffected by the Affordable Care Act of 2010.

Managed care isintended to reduce unnecessary health care costs through a variety of mechanisms, including: economic incentives for physicians and patients to select less costly forms of care; programs for reviewing the medical necessity of specific services; increased beneficiary cost sharing; controls on inpatient admissions and lengths of stay; the establishment of cost-sharing incentives for outpatient surgery; selective contracting with health care providers; and the intensive management of high-cost health care cases. The programs may be provided in a variety of settings, such as Health Maintenance Organizations and Preferred Provider Organizations

Managed Competition

A purchasing strategy to obtain maximum value for consumers and employers, using rules for competition derived from microeconomic principles. A sponsor (either an employer, a governmental entity, or a purchasing cooperative), acting on behalf of a large group of subscribers, structures and adjusts the market to overcome attempts by insurers to avoid price competition. The sponsor establishes rules of equity, selects participating plans, manages the enrollment process, creates price-elastic demand, and manages risk selection.

Minimally invasive surgery

In minimally invasive surgery, doctors use various techniques to operate with less damage to the body than with open surgery. In general, minimally invasive surgery is associated with less pain, a shorter hospital stay and fewer complications. Laparoscopic surgery and robotic surgery are examples.

MPM or PMS

Medical practice management (MPM) software is a collection of computerized services used by healthcare professionals and administration to streamline day-to-day tasks within medical practice and improve the efficiency of operations and quality of patient care. PMS is the same thing and stands for patient management software

National Health Mission (NHM)

The National Health Mission (NHM) was launched by the government of India in 2005 subsuming the National Rural Health Mission and

National Urban Health Mission. It was further extended in March 2018, to continue until March 2020. It is headed by Mission Director and monitored by National Level Monitors appointed by the Government of India Rural Health Mission (NRHM) and the recently launched National Urban Health Mission (NUHM). Main program components include Health System Strengthening in rural and urban areas- Reproductive-Maternal- Neonatal-Child and Adolescent Health, and Communicable and Non-Communicable Diseases (RMNCH+A). NHM envisages achievement of universal access to equitable, affordable and quality health care services that are accountable and responsive to the needs of the people.

Programs under NHM

Reproductive, Maternal, Newborn, Child And Adolescent Health: RMNCH+A approach has been launched in 2013 and it essentially looks to address the major causes of mortality among women and children

Rashtriya Bal Swasthya Karyakram: From survival to healthy survival

India Newborn Action Plan: INAP is India's committed response to the Global Every Newborn Action Plan, launched in June 2014 at the 67th World Health Assembly

Janani Shishu Suraksha Karyakaram (JSSK): JSSK launched on 1st of June, 2011 is an initiative to assure free services to all pregnant women and sick neonates accessing public health institutions.

Rashtriya Kishor Swasthya Karyakram: The Ministry of Health & Family Welfare has launched a health program for adolescents, in the age group of10-19 years.

NATIONAL HEALTHCARE INNOVATIONS PORTAL: nhinp.org

MERA ASPATAAL: https://meraaspataal.nhp.gov.in//about_us

Out-of-pocket payment

An out-of-pocket expense is a payment you make with your own money, even if you are reimbursed later. In terms of health insurance, out-of-pocket expenses are your share of covered healthcare costs, including the money you pay for deductibles, copays, and coinsurance.

Patient-centered medical home

The patient-centered medical home (PCMH) model is an approach to delivering high-quality, cost-effective primary care. Using a patient-centered, culturally appropriate, and team-based approach, the PCMH model coordinates patient care across the health system.

PHR

A personal health record (PHR) is a health record where health data and other information related to the care of a patient is maintained by the patient.

POC

Point of care

POS (point-of-service plan)

a hybrid of an HMO and a PPO; offering an open-access model that may assign members to a primary care physician and usually provides partial coverage for out-of-network services.

PPACA

Patient Protection and Affordable Care Act - The goals of the PPACA are to ensure more people have health insurance, reduce the cost of health care, and improve how patients get care. The final modified version of the law is referred to simply as the Affordable Care Act or "Obamacare."

PPO

A type of health plan that contracts with medical providers, such as hospitals and doctors, to create a network of participating providers. You pay less if you use providers that belong to the plan's network.

Primary care

Primary care is the day-to-day healthcare given by a healthcare provider. Typically, this provider acts as the first contact and principal point of continuing care for patients within a healthcare system and coordinates other specialist care that the patient may need

QALY

Quality-adjusted life years: a generic measure of disease burden, including both the quality and the quantity of life lived. It is used in economic evaluation to assess the value of medical interventions. One QALY equates to one year in perfect health.

Quaternary care

Quaternary care is an advanced level of specialized care delivered in a hospital, e.g. bone marrow transplantation

Secondary care

Secondary care is when you see a specialist such as an oncologist or endocrinologist.

Solution shop

These "shops" are businesses that are structured to diagnose and solve unstructured problems. Solution shops deliver value primarily through the people they employ, experts who draw upon their intuition and analytical and problem-solving skills to diagnose the cause of complicated problems.

Tele-health

tele-health refers to the provision of remote clinical services, via real-time two-way communication between the patient and the healthcare provider, using electronic audio and visual means.

Telemedicine

Same as tele-health

Tertiary care

Tertiary care refers to specialized care in a hospital setting, such as dialysis or heart surgery.

Third-party administrator (TPA)

A third-party administrator is a company that provides operational services such as claims processing and employee benefits management under contract to another company. Insurance companies and self-insured companies often outsource their claims processing to third parties. Thus, such companies are often called third-party claims administrators.

Value-adding process business

Business that transforms inputs into outputs of greater value through process excellence. For example, focused value-adding process hospitals and clinics can deliver care at prices that are 60 per cent lower than those at non-focused institutions

Value-based healthcare

Value-based healthcare is a payment system that compensates healthcare providers in accordance with the quality of care provided to their patients

Wellness

"Wellness is a state of complete physical, mental, and social well-being, and not merely the absence of disease or infirmity." – The World Health Organization

TABLES AND COMMENTARY

Tables start on Page 64

DEMOGRAPHICS IMPACTING HEALTHCARE

Table 1: India's population is aging rapidly. By 2050, there will be 320 million people over 60 years old.

After China, India will have the largest number of people 60+ years old by 2050, which will be three times the number in the US at that time. Since 60+ year-olds consume a disproportionately high share of healthcare, this can be expected to put huge pressure on the supply of healthcare that the aging population will need.

Table 2: Life expectancy in India has increased in the last three decades with mixed consequences

Past increases in life expectancy were mainly due to drastic reductions in infant mortality, maternal mortality, and mortality from communicable diseases. In the future, life expectancy is expected to increase due to treatments that prolong life. Unfortunately, India has the highest gap between healthy life years and total life years, which means that many Indians at the end of life are in poor health. Therefore, any increases in life expectancy without improving health status will only magnify the impact of the end-of-life disease burden. Many more Indians will die old, poor, and sick if NCDs and diseases of aging are not prevented and also managed adequately.

Table 3: Indians lose 43 days every year due to disability.

Table 4: By 2050, the notional cost to the economy of the top 6 NCDs will exceed India's total health spending

Table 5: By 2030, NCDs will account for close to 70% of all DALYs lost.

Despite a youthful population, Indians already lose a very high number of days due to disability. This is despite a relatively low contribution of NCDs to disability. Days lost due to disability are higher in countries with NCDs. As the prevalence of NCDs accelerates from 58% now to 80% (comparable to developed nations), NCDs will account for 80% of DALYs. This will severely impact productivity and reduce incomes. Cancers and mental disorders will emerge as major contributors to the NCD burden. Mental health is relatively neglected in health programmes, and as families become smaller and disperse, the mentally ill will pose a significant burden unless provision is made for their appropriate care when their family members are unwilling to take care of them.

GDP GROWTH, HEALTHCARE, and HEALTH EQUITY

Table 6: India is projected to have the fastest-growing GDP per capita in PPP terms by 2050.

Table 7: Even as India moves toward becoming the second-largest economy, widening income inequality poses a threat to equity in healthcare.

Table 8: On the UHC service coverage index (UHC score), India ranks 121 overall with a score of 61.

Table 9: Despite economic tailwinds, growth in healthcare spending is slowing.

India's per capita GDP will rise from 1/10th of the US today to 1/3rd of the US by 2050. Given that India's population will be 5X that of the US, this is a huge expansion in absolute GDP. If India followed the US model of healthcare, then a substantial fraction of the expansion in GDP (~20%) will go toward healthcare, reducing the capital available for other investments needed in a developed economy. If India can contain the allocation of resources to healthcare at 6%, it will provide enormous headroom for the investments needed to put the economy on a firm footing through investments in education, livelihoods, innovation, and infrastructure. Key areas of investment that can deliver good healthcare while containing runaway inflation in healthcare costs include:

a.   Information technology that delivers a comprehensive health record for every citizen;

b.   Health Economic Zones (just like SEZ) to house focused healthcare factories for elective procedures (which can also attract patients from developed countries) and

c.   Training of health workers to create a skilled pool that can work globally.

Economic growth is a given; however, the economic surplus is not being shared fairly across the population. The richest 1% in India can afford care anywhere in the world. The richest 10% are protected by insurance. It is the middle 40% and the bottom 50% that are worst affected by inequity in access to healthcare. While the bottom 50% are obvious candidates for social security schemes, the middle 40% cannot be abandoned since their precarious incomes and modest savings mean that a single catastrophic illness event can push them into poverty. Out-of-pocket expenditure already accounts for more than 50% of spending on healthcare in India, which is unsustainable. UHC must, therefore, guarantee coverage for both the middle 40% and bottom 50%. Countries with high out-of-pocket expenditures also fare poorly on the UHC score, indicating that when a healthcare safety net is unavailable through UHC, out-of-pocket expenditures grow and impoverish those who have the misfortune of experiencing a serious illness. India's low UHC score is largely due to access issues that must be corrected as an early priority as part of UHC. Despite satisfactory economic growth that should give room for the government to allocate more fiscal resources to healthcare, growth in spend on healthcare per capita is actually declining. The flattening of out-of-pocket spends may be due to a combination of government spends targeting the poorer classes and the inability of the bottom 50% to take on any further increase in such expenditure. There is healthy growth in hospital care but flat or negative growth in diagnostic and pharmacy spends. This may be due to a shift in OPD spends to hospitals. Decline in OPD spends outside hospitals is a factor that can drive increased hospitalization rates since hospitals use their OPDs as catchment areas to recruit patients. It also reflects poorly on the availability and use of primary care services.

HEALTHCARE INFRA AND HEALTHCARE WORKERS

Table 10: State of health infrastructure in 2012

Table 11: Availability of beds per 1000 populations varies widely across India

Table 12: India has a shortage of doctors in rural areas and an even greater shortage of nurses

On top of the relative under-capacity in many areas, India's healthcare is crippled by poor-quality infrastructure, as revealed in these tables. The fact that 25.5% of sub-centers lack water or power or both is a stunning revelation of the apathy of administration toward providing basic needs. There is also wide variability between states in the availability of hospital beds. Among the large states, some like Tamil Nadu and Karnataka do very well. On the other hand, major states like Uttar Pradesh and Madhya Pradesh are grossly under resourced. If we accounted for the fact that much of this capacity is in or near urban centers, the lack of access among the rural population in UP and MP is even more stark. On the human resources front, India has a less talked about but even more consequential shortage of nurses. Building the physical infrastructure can be managed, but training sufficient numbers of nurses and other categories of healthcare workers will call for a drastic change in both the scale and type of training given in order to produce the required numbers in a decade or less.

INSURANCE

Table 13: Growth in insurance coverage

The fastest growth in coverage is in employer-sponsored private insurance. Government social health insurance and self-paid insurance have grown relatively modestly despite the enormous informal work sector in the Indian economy. Many such Indians are left to fend for themselves without adequate protection from a Government safety net or through affordable self-purchased insurance policies. These are the people who will benefit the most from UHC, and they are a big chunk of the population.

WASTE, FRAUD AND ERROR IN HEALTHCARE (WaFEr)

Table 14: Estimates of waste in US healthcare spending, by category in 2011 (USD Billion)

The total waste (midpoint estimate) is in the region of USD 910 Billion or 34% of total healthcare spending. Corresponding figures are not available for India, although it is likely to be the same or perhaps even higher, since private consumption (fee for service) accounts for a significant chunk of healthcare spending, and it is the place where WaFEr is magnified. Unless this is squeezed out of the healthcare economy, any increased spending on UHC may simply add to the waste of resources with only marginal benefits to the poor in terms of better healthcare.

HEALTHCARE START-UPs

Table 15: India's healthcare start-up ecosystem

Most players are in the services space. India needs more start-ups developing new product solutions in healthcare. This can happen if we had safe spaces for such start-ups to emerge such as the Health Innovation Parks mentioned in the section on Health Technology.

SOURCES FOR TABLES

1. Institute of Health Metrics and Evaluation (IHME) (https://www.healthdata.org/); LE is Life Expectancy in years, HLE is Healthy Life Expectancy in years;

2. https://unstats.un.org/unsd/snaama/Index (National Accounts-Main aggregates database of the United Nations) and https://unstats.un.org/unsd/snaama/Downloads

3. https://data.worldbank.org/indicator/SH.XPD.CHEX.GD.ZS

4. PwC Report Feb 2017-The World in 2050

5. World Inequality Report 2022-Data for Philippines not available

6. World Inequality Database (https://wid.world/)

7. National Institute of Public Finance and Policy-Nov 1992-Health Expenditures in India

8. National Health Accounts Estimates for India 2013-14 through 2018-19

9. www.who.int/news-room/fact-sheets/detail/universal-health-coverage-(uhc)

10. Handbook on Insurance Statistics-2021-22, www.irdai.gov.in

11. Niti Aayog Report-Nov 2019, Health Systems for a new India

12. National Health Profile 2018. 13th and 2023, 14th Issue

13. CDDEP Report-Apr 2020, Statewise estimates of hospital beds

14. OECD Health Statistics 2020-Frequently requested data

15. Population Pyramid (population in 2019)

16. Health Policy Brief: Reducing Waste in Health Care," *Health Affairs*, December 13, 2012.

17. Donald M Berwick and Andrew D Hackbarth, "Eliminating waste in US healthcare, JAMA 307, no 14 (Apr 11, 2012):1513-6, Copyright 2012, American Medical Assn

Table 1: India's population is ageing rapidly. By 2050, there will be 320 Million people over 60 years old

| S. No | Country | Population (Mil) | | Increase in Population | Average Age (yrs) | | Share of 60+ | | | | 60+ added |
| | | | | | | | 2019 | | 2050 | | 2019-50 |
		2019	2050	2019-50	2019	2050	Share	Nos (Mil)	Share	Nos (mil)	Nos (Mil)
1	China	1433	1402	-31	37.2	45.6	16.8%	241	34.6%	485	244
2	India	1366	1639	273	30.2	38.0	9.8%	134	19.5%	320	186
3	USA	328	379	51	38.9	42.7	22.4%	73	28.1%	106	33
4	Indonesia	260	331	72	30.9	38.0	9.7%	25	21.0%	70	44
5	Mexico	125	155	30	31.1	39.6	10.9%	14	22.5%	35	21
6	UK	67	74	7	40.5	44.3	24.1%	16	31.6%	23	7
7	Bangladesh	159	193	34	29.2	39.6	7.7%	12	21.8%	42	30
8	Nigeria	215	401	187	22.1	25.5	4.5%	10	6.3%	25	16
9	Philippines	112	145	33	28.2	35.6	8.3%	9	16.5%	24	15
10	Canada	37	46	9	40.8	45.5	24.2%	9	31.7%	15	6

Table 2: Life expectancy in India has increased in the last 3 decades with mixed consequences

S. No	Country	Life expectancy (Males)			Life expectancy (females)			LE	HLE
								All	
		1990	2019	2050	1990	2019	2050	2019	2019
1	China	66.9	74.5	79.0	70.7	79.9	84.0	76.9	68.7
2	India	58.9	67.8	74.0	60.4	70.2	77.5	69.7	60.6
3	USA	72.1	76.1	79.0	79.0	81.1	83.0	78.8	68.5
4	Indonesia	62.4	69.2	74.0	65.4	73.9	79.0	71.7	62.7
5	Mexico	68.6	72.6	78.0	74.3	78.5	82.0	75.7	67.4
6	UK	72.9	79.2	82.5	78.5	82.7	85.5	81.2	71.0
7	Bangladesh	57.3	71.8	78.5	59.5	74.6	81.0	73.9	64.1
8	Nigeria	54.0	62.8	74.0	57.1	65.8	77.5	55.2	53.6
9	Philippines	64.6	66.6	72.0	71.4	73.1	77.5	71.0	63.6
10	Canada	74.1	79.9	82.0	80.6	84.0	86.0	82.5	73.0
1	LE is Life Expectancy in years, HLE is Healthy Life Expectancy in years; The difference between LE and HLE is the number of years people will live, but with disabilities								

Table 3: Indians lose 43 days every year due to disability

S.No	Country	DALYs	NCD DALYs	NCD share of DALYs	YLD	Days lost per year due to disability
		Mil	Mil	NCD	Mil	Days
1	China	382	325	85.0%	154	39
2	India	468	271	57.9%	160	43
3	USA	111	96	86.4%	53	59
4	Indonesia	77	56	72.4%	26	37
5	Mexico	34	25	73.5%	13	38
6	UK	20	17	86.3%	10	54
7	Bangladesh	43	28	65.0%	16	37
8	Nigeria	116	31	26.7%	20	34
9	Philippines	33	21	64.2%	11	36
10	Canada	10	9	90.0%	5	50

YLL - Years of life lost due to premature death

YLD - Years lived with disability (years lived in states of less than full health)

DALY = YLL + YLD

Table 4: By 2050, the notional cost to the economy of the top 6 NCDs will exceed India's total health spending

S. No	Summary for India	2019		2050	CAGR
	Population (millions)	1366		1639	0.59%
	Total DALYs (Millions)	468		487	0.10%
	DALYs from NCD	271		397	1.20%
	NCD share of DALYs	57.9%		81.5%	1.10%
	GDP in $ B (Nominal)	2832		13119	5.07%
	Health spend/ Capita $	57		150	3.17%
	Total Health Spend $B	78		246	3.78%
	Share of GDP	2.7%		1.9%	

S. No	Disease category	2019		2050	
		DALYs-Mil	Cost in $ B	DALYs-Mil	Cost in $ B
1	Cancers	27	56.4	51	405.9
2	Cardiovascular	65	134.6	96	766.3
3	Injuries	54	112.0	43	344.2
4	Chronic Respiratory	29	60.5	42	335.1
5	Diabetes and Kidney	20	42.1	44	352.0
6	Musculoskeletal disorders	23	46.6	39	312.2
	Total	**218**	**452.2**	**314**	**2516**

Table 5: By 2030, NCDs will account for close to 70% of all DALYs lost

S. No	Disease category	Decadal Change				Estimated	DALYs in 2030		Ranking
		1990-99	2000-09	2010-18	2019-30		per 100k	Total-Mil	of DALYs
A	**Deficiencies/ Infections**								
1	Nutritional Deficiencies	-41.2%	-32.7%	-21.7%	-21.7%		924	14	15
2	Maternal Disorders	-23.3%	-45.1%	-40.0%	-40.0%		122	2	20
3	Neonatal Disorders	-24.1%	-28.2%	-36.7%	-36.7%		1965	30	6
4	Malaria/Tropical Diseases	-53.5%	-35.1%	-39.5%	-39.5%		265	4	19
5	Enteric Infections	-31.5%	-40.1%	-43.0%	-43.0%		1026	16	14
6	HIV/AIDS/STD	273.5%	-11.2%	-61.8%	-61.8%		95	1	20
7	Other infectious diseases	-38.4%	-47.1%	-59.3%	-59.3%		306	5	17
8	Respiratory Infections	-31.6%	-37.8%	-35.1%	-35.1%		1667	25	10
B	**Non Communicable**								
9	Cancers	4.9%	4.4%	17.0%	20.7%		2365	36	3
10	Cardiovascular (CVD)	1.7%	3.6%	7.8%	9.5%		5115	77	1
11	Chronic Respiratory	-1.1%	-0.5%	6.8%	8.3%		2275	34	4
12	Digestive Diseases	-1.5%	-9.4%	-7.4%	-7.4%		1230	19	12
13	Diabetes and Kidney	21.6%	11.3%	23.5%	28.7%		1880	28	6
14	Musculoskeletal disorders	-2.3%	14.3%	14.0%	17.1%		1896	29	5
15	Neurological disorders	-0.5%	0.3%	8.0%	9.8%		1188	18	11
16	Mental Disorders	6.1%	-2.2%	4.4%	5.4%		1660	25	8
17	Substance use disorders	8.2%	-5.6%	0.7%	0.8%		292	4	17
18	Other non communicable	-13.2%	-10.0%	-12.5%	-12.5%		1704	26	9
19	Sense Organ Disorders	7.0%	4.9%	9.3%	11.4%		1072	16	13
20	Skin related	-0.9%	-3.0%	-2.7%	-2.7%		488	7	16

Table 5: By 2030, NCDs will account for close to 70% of all DALYs lost							
C	**Injuries**						
21	Injuries	-6.6%	-13.4%	-13.9%	-13.9%	3317	50	2
S. No	**Summary**	**Decadal Change**			**Projected**	**2030**		
		1990-2000	2000-2010	2010-2019	2019-2030	per 100 K	Total Mil	Share
A	**Deficiencies/ Infections**	-31.4%	-35.9%	-39.8%	-38.1%	6371	97	20.6%
B	**Non Communicable**	0.2%	0.5%	5.8%	8.6%	21164	321	68.6%
C	**Injuries**	-6.6%	-13.4%	-13.9%	-13.9%	3317	50	10.8%
	Total	**-20.0%**	**-20.3%**	**-15.9%**	**-8.3%**	**30852**	**467**	

Table 6: India projected to have the fastest growing GDP per Capita in PPP terms by 2050						
S. No	Country	GDP per capita ($)		GDP-PPP* per capita ($)		CAGR
		2019	2050	2019	2050	GDP-PPP
1	China	10008	25620	16299	41725	3.0%
2	India	2073	8004	6974	26924	5.1%
3	USA	65162	89979	65162	89979	1.5%
4	Indonesia	4312	10655	12840	31728	3.8%
5	Mexico	10160	21381	21041	44277	3.1%
6	UK	42857	63090	49286	72554	1.5%
7	Bangladesh	2203	5640	6202	15876	3.7%
8	Nigeria	2086	4511	5009	10835	4.6%
9	Philippines	3363	8625	8965	22993	3.9%
10	Canada	47260	60084	53123	67538	1.5%

***GDP-PPP is GDP expressed in terms of purchasing power parity**

Table 7: Even as India moves towards becoming the second largest economy, widening income inequality poses a threat to equity in healthcare

S. No	Country	GDP	GDP-PPP	Top	Top	Middle	Bottom	Top	Top	Middle	Bottom
		per Cap ($)	per Cap ($)	1%	10%	40%	50%	1%	10%	40%	50%
		2019	2019	Share of total income				GDP Per Capita-PPP $			
1	China	10008	16299	14.0%	41.7%	44.0%	14.4%	228181	67965	17929	4694
2	India	2073	6974	21.7%	57.1%	29.7%	13.1%	151328	39820	5178	1827
3	USA	65162	65162	18.8%	45.5%	41.2%	13.3%	1225038	296485	67116	17333
4	Indonesia	4312	12840	18.3%	48.0%	39.6%	12.4%	234973	61632	12712	3184
5	Mexico	10160	21041	26.1%	57.4%	33.5%	9.2%	549166	120774	17622	3872
6	UK	42857	49286	12.7%	35.7%	44.0%	20.4%	625929	175950	54214	20109
7	Bangladesh	2203	6202	16.3%	42.9%	40.0%	17.1%	101095	26607	3675	2121
8	Nigeria	2086	5009	11.6%	42.7%	41.8%	15.5%	58108	21390	5235	1553
9	Philippines	3363	8965	NA	NA	NA	NA	NA	NA	NA	NA
10	Canada	47726	53123	10.5%	30.8%	45.4%	23.8%	557795	163620	60295	25287

Table 8: On the UHC service coverage index (UHC score), India ranks 121 overall with a score of 61

| S. No | Country | percentage of HH* Spending on Healthcare | | | | OOPE** | UHC |
| | | >10% HH Income | | >25% of HH Income | | % | Score |
		2000	2017	2000	2017	2019	2019
1	China	12.3%	24.0%	3.0%	9.2%	35.5%	82
2	India	15.4%	17.3%	3.1%	6.5%	63.0%	61
3	USA	5.8%	4.5%	1.0%	0.7%	10.9%	83
4	Indonesia	2.6%	4.3%	0.3%	0.9%	35.1%	59
5	Mexico	3.6%	1.6%	0.7%	0.2%	41.6%	74
6	UK	2.0%	2.2%	0.3%	0.4%	16.5%	88
7	Bangladesh	14.9%	24.4%	4.8%	8.5%	78.5%	51
8	Nigeria	22.9%	15.8%	10.6%	4.1%	83.0%	44
9	Philippines	2.8%	6.3%	0.6%	1.4%	53.7%	55
10	Canada	3.0%	3.8%	0.5%	0.8%	14.8%	89

*** HH is household**
****OOPE is out of pocket expenditure on healthcare**

Table 9: Despite economic tailwinds, growth in healthcare spending is slowing

No	Description	2013-14	2014-15	2015-16	2016-17	2017-18	2018-19	2019-20	CAGR
1	GDP-Per Capita (INR)	89796	98405	107342	118489	130061	142328	151431	9.10%
2	Healthcare spending-Per Capita (INR)	3250	3445	3737	4028	3708	3955	4293	4.70%
3	Health care spend/GDP per capita (%)	3.6	3.5	3.5	3.4	2.9	2.8	2.8	
	SPENDING BY CATEGORY	**ALL FIGURES BELOW IN INR CR**							
1	National Health Expenditure	421194	451286	495190	539371	501760	540246	593659	5.90%
2	Government Health Expenditure	97866	107975	127736	145757	166377	186025	209381	13.50%
3	Private Health Expenditure	323328	343311	367454	393614	335383	354221	384278	2.92%
4	Out of pocket	290932	302425	320211	340916	276532	287573	308727	1.00%
5	Not for profit providers	6782	8588	9196	9028	8671	9367	9099	6.67%
6	Employer paid	10203	14543	16032	16327	17092	18064	18478	10.40%
7	Health insurance	15413	17755	22013	27339	33087	39215	45877	19.90%
a	- Employer provided	8017	8899	11621	14718	17757	21676	25881	21.60%
b	- Self-purchased	7330	8772	10353	12584	15291	17526	19957	18.20%
c	- Community insurance	66	84	39	37	39	13	39	-8.39%
	CONSUMPTION BY CATEGORY								
1	Hospitals	134888	181628	199544	221479	230552	248702	271773	12.40%
a	- Government	45545	64685	70954	80397	85287	93689	102579	14.50%
b	- Private	89343	116943	128590	141082	145265	155013	169194	11.20%
2	Diagnostic labs	28035	21058	22715	24058	20324	21162	22765	-3.40%
3	Pharmacies	150773	131100	138853	151397	117139	122720	132452	-2.10%

Table 10: State of Health infrastructure in 2012

No.	Description	Numbers	Share
	Hospitals		
1	Total hospital beds	1373000	
2	Beds per 1000 population	1.08	
3	Private Sector hospital beds	833000	60.7%
4	Public Sector hospital beds	540000	39.3%
5	Functional Beds	853100	62.1%
a	Private Sector	583100	
b	Public Sector	270000	
6	Top 20 cities functional beds	570170	41.5%
a	Private Sector	408170	
b	Public Sector	162000	
6	Other Cities functional beds	282930	20.6%
a	Private Sector	174930	
b	Public Sector	108000	
	Primary health centres		
a	Subcentres without an Auxiliary Nurse Midwife		3.2%
b	PHCs without doctors		3.8%
c	Subcentres without water and/or power		25.5%
d	PHCs without water and/or power		10.7%
e	Subcentres without motorable road access		6.6%
f	PHCs without motorable road access		5.8%

Table 11: Availability of beds per 1000 population varies significantly across India

S. No	State	Govt. Beds	Private Beds	Total Beds	Popn Mil	Beds/1000
1	Uttar Pradesh	76260	130733	206993	238.0	0.87
2	Maharashtra	51446	88194	139640	123.0	1.14
3	Bihar	12019	20604	32623	125.0	0.26
4	West Bengal	78566	134686	213252	100.0	2.13
5	Andhra Pradesh	23138	39665	62803	54.0	1.16
6	Madhya Pradesh	28839	49439	78278	85.0	0.92
7	Rajasthan	31848	54597	86445	81.0	1.07
8	Tamil Nadu	77532	132913	210445	76.0	2.77
9	Karnataka	69865	119770	189635	68.4	2.77
10	Gujarat	32280	55338	87618	64.0	1.37
11	Odisha	18519	31747	50266	46.0	1.09
12	Telangana	20983	35971	56954	39.0	1.46
13	Kerala	38004	65150	103154	36.0	2.87
14	Jharkhand	10784	18487	29271	39.0	0.75
15	Assam	17142	29387	46529	36.0	1.29
16	Punjab	17933	30743	48676	30.0	1.62
17	Haryana	11240	19269	30509	28.1	1.09
18	Chhattisgarh	9412	16135	25547	24.9	1.03
19	Delhi	24383	41800	66183	20.1	3.29
20	Jammu and Kashmir	11651	19973	31624	14.0	2.26
21	Uttarakhand	8512	14592	23104	10.5	2.20
22	Himachal Pradesh	12399	21256	33655	7.2	4.71
23	Tripura	4417	7572	11989	3.9	3.11
24	Meghalaya	4457	7641	12098	2.8	4.32
25	Manipur	1427	2446	3873	2.5	1.55
26	Nagaland	1880	3223	5103	2.4	2.17
27	Goa	3013	5165	8178	2.0	4.05
28	Chandigarh	778	1334	2112	1.8	1.19
29	Puducherry	3569	6118	9687	1.4	7.02
30	Arunachal Pradesh	2404	4121	6525	1.3	4.94
31	Mizoram	1997	3423	5420	1.1	5.07
32	Sikkim	1560	2674	4234	0.7	6.51
33	A & N Island	1075	1843	2918	0.6	5.31
34	D & N Haveli	589	1010	1599	0.4	3.72
35	Lakshadweep	300	514	814	0.1	10.18
	Total	**710221**	**1217532**	**1927753**	**1365.9**	**1.41**

Table 12: India has a shortage of doctors and an even greater shortage of nurses					
S. No	Country	Doctors	Nurses	Beds	ICU Beds
		per 1000 population			
1	China	2.20	3.00	5.20	0.036
2	India	0.74	1.80	1.41	0.070
3	USA	2.60	15.70	2.77	0.258
4	Indonesia	0.62	3.90	1.18	0.050
5	Mexico	2.40	2.90	1.00	0.033
6	UK	3.00	8.50	2.44	0.105
7	Bangladesh	0.66	0.50	0.85	0.008
8	Nigeria	0.50	1.50	0.20	0.003
9	Philippines	0.80	5.40	1.00	0.040
10	Canada	2.44	11.00	2.58	0.129

Table 13: Growth in insurance coverage

A. Government policies - Social Health Insurance

No	Period	No of policies	Persons Mil	Premium Rs. Cr	Premium/ Person (Rs)
1	2013-14	32087	155	2082	134
2	2021-22	62000	307	6076	198
	CAGR		**8.9%**	**14.3%**	**5.0%**

B. Employer sponsored private insurance / Group policies

No	Period	Policies Mil	Persons Mil	Premium Rs. Cr	Premium/ Person (Rs)
1	2013-14	0.19	34	8057	2370
2	2021-22	0.7	162	36890	2277
	CAGR		**21.5%**	**20.9%**	**-0.4%**

C. Individual purchased-retail policies

No.	Period	Policies Mil	Persons Mil	Premium Rs. Cr	Premium/ Person (Rs)
1	2013-14	9.8	27	7355	2724
2	2021-22	21.9	52	30085	5786
	CAGR		**8.5%**	**19.2%**	**9.9%**

D. Total Insurance policies

No.	Period	Policies Mil	Persons Mil	Premium Rs. Cr	Premium/ Person (Rs)
1	2013-14	10.02	216	17494	810
2	2021-22	22.60	521	73051	1402
	CAGR		**11.6%**	**19.6%**	**7.1%**

Table 14: Estimates of waste in US Healthcare spending, by category in 2011 ($ Billion)							
S. No	Category	Cost to Medicare and Medicaid			Total cost to US Healthcare		
		Low	Mid point	High	Low	Mid point	High
1	Failures of care delivery	26	36	45	102	128	158
2	Failures of care coordination	21	30	39	25	35	45
3	Overtreatment	67	77	87	158	192	226
4	Administrative complexity	16	36	56	107	248	389
5	Pricing failures	36	56	77	84	131	178
	Subtotal (excl fraud/abuse)	166	235	304	476	734	996
	%age of total health spend	6%	9%	11%	18%	27%	37%
6	Fraud and abuse	30	64	98	82	177	272
	Total (incl fraud/abuse)	197	300	402	558	910	1263
	Percentage of total health spend				21%	34%	47%

Table 15: India's healthcare start-up ecosystem

Archetype	Business model	Legacy Players	Disruptors	Disruption
HEALTHCARE SERVICES	Branded hospital chains	Apollo, Fortis	Pristyn	Capacity aggregation and resale
	Focused chronic care	Dr. Mohan's Diabetes Specialities	Wellthy, Sugar.Fit, CredoHealth, BeatO	Tech solutions to managing metabolic disorders
	Telehealth	Teleconsult (phone based: Dial 104)	Tricog, CloudPhysician	Delivered remotely
	Diagnostic laboratories	Dr. Lal, Metropolis	Redcliffe Labs	Technology empowered
	Home healthcare	Nightingale	Portea	Large scale with larger footprint
	Pharmacies	MedPlus, Apollo Pharmacy	1 mg, Netmeds	Online, home delivery, and discounted prices
TECHNOLOGY	Services - IT	TCS, Wipro		
	Products - IT		Practo	Disruption by creating a product
	Products		Forus, Dozee,	
FINANCIAL INTERMEDIARIES	Insurance	NIA, OIC, UIC, NIC	Kenko General Insurance, Even Health	More OPD Coverage
	Broking	Marsh, Towers Watson, Aon	Plum, Onsurity	Tech driven, primary care benefits
	TPA	Mediassist, Vidal Health	Claimsbuddy	Hospitals as clients
	Loans		BajajFinserv	Instant discharge
	Crowdfunding		Milaap, Impact Guru, Ketto	OOP funding
ECOSYSTEM SUPPORT	Supply chain	Traditional distributors	MedikaBazaar, Aknamed, Stratmed	Online marketplaces

ABOUT THE AUTHORS

Swami Subramaniam is a physician-scientist who spent most of his career in the biopharmaceutical industry. He co-founded Aurigene Discovery Technologies, headed business development for a Danish biotech, and spent several years in in R&D in Merck (MSD) and Abbott Nutrition. He currently heads - Ignite Life Science Foundation, a science philanthropy with the mission - "Making Science Work for India".

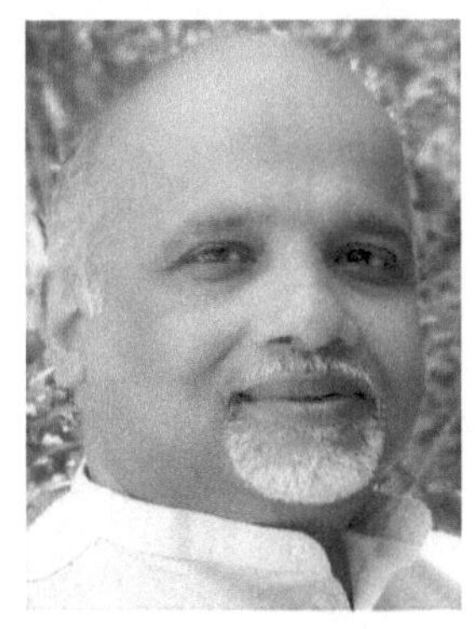

He is the author of two books – Mastering Sleep, the science behind sleeping well and Healing Hands – the biography of a plastic surgeon who set up the worlds largest hand injury service at a Government hsopital in Chennai. He can be reached at swami2m@gmail.com

Aparajithan Srivathsan has over 3 decades built world class solutions for India's healthcare needs with a ringside view of private healthcare, health insurance and health-tech. Srivathsan is a hospital strategist and health systems tinkerer. He believes in the ability of technology to democratize access to healthcare and the need for tech-enabled frontline community health workers to take healthcare into the community. He believes in the promise of India as a hub for global

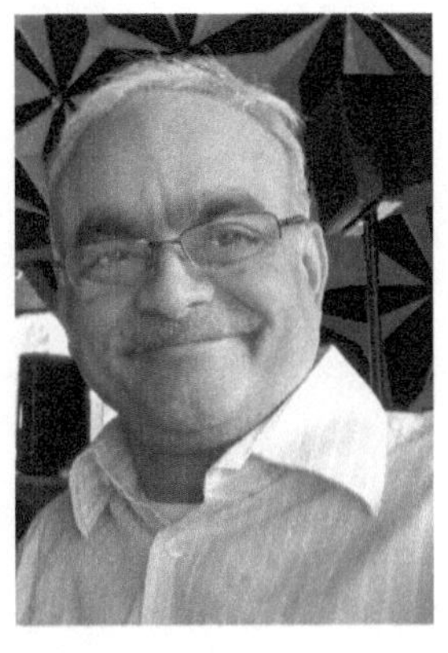

medicine and innovator of solutions that can be applied to healthcare globally. He can be reached at srivathsan.aparajithan@gmail.com.